Adventures in Walking
From the Couch to 5K

Adventures in Walking
From the Couch to 5K

Mandy Jo Rindhage
2018

First Printing: 2018

ISBN #: 978-0-359-07036-7

Lulu Press, Inc.
 627 Davis Drive, Suite 300
Morrisville, NC 27560

Ordering Information:

 Discounts available on bulk quantity purchases by corporations, associations, educators, and others. For details, contact the publisher at the above listed address.

 U.S. trade bookstores and wholesalers: Please contact Mandy Jo Rindhage   email   mandyjo@mandyjo.us.

Dedication

I have a lot of people to thank:

Rick Squires, my boyfriend and my rock for being there and being supportive

Jenn Paul, my friend and model for the exercises

Vickie Hohauser, my friend, former trainee and editor

Martha Andrus, my friend and reader

The Crim Training Program, where I got my start

The Brooksie Training Program for welcoming me into their program after the Crim

All of my former trainees and group co-leaders

My boys, Bryan Rindhage & Bradley Suwienski

My parents, Fred & Mary Lou Rindhage, for being supportive

Larry Suwienski, my ex & late husband for working so well with me with the boys during training through the years

Aspiring Writers Association of America (AWAOA), so many friends and wonderful insights for my writing

All of my supportive friends and family

Contents

Preface

Have you thought of taking up some form of exercise?

Have you decided that you would like to do a race?

Have your friends been doing races and keep asking you to join them?

Have you been discouraged by people telling you that you have to run?

Have you been looking for something different to read?

If you have answered yes to any or all of these questions, you have found a book that will help you get moving, complete a race, join your friends, give you encouragement to walk, and will be a different book for you to read.

After reading many training books, most of which were aimed towards runners and not walkers, I wanted a book that would encourage the walker to continue walking.

While working with walking trainees through a couple of training programs I came across the same questions year after year from trainees. Then it came to me, I should be writing all these answers down. However, I didn't want it to be just another training manual. This book is not just another training manual. It's a fictional story that includes training for walking your first 5K (3.1 mile) race.

I won't tell you how it ends, but I can guarantee you that it does not include running.

Introduction

Andrea is a divorced mother of twin five-year-old boys entering her 30's. She ran cross-country back in high school but has not done any running since then and has put on a few pounds. She has been feeling sluggish and wants to begin a healthier lifestyle, i.e. lose weight and begin an exercise routine. Also, she wants to be a good influence on her boys. Andrea finds a training program that will help her incorporate exercise into her life.

Throughout Andrea's first journey from the couch to a 5K race you get to train with her and see how she handles training with twins, when the weather does not cooperate, her ex is late and more. You will find her training schedule, exercises, recipes and some of the locations where she trains at and visits.

Train along with Andrea and reach your goal of completing a 5K.

Happy reading and walking!

Chapter 1: Let's Get Started

It's a warm and sunny early spring morning with the birds chirping out the window. Andrea is eating breakfast with her twins, Cooper and Carson, in the dining room of their townhouse. The boys are chattering away with the flat screen television playing their favorite cartoon, Scooby Doo. A commercial comes on for a beginner's training program to walk a 5K.

Andrea thinks to herself, *I would love to lose 25 pounds, this would be a great start. Plus, I ran cross country in high school, I could walk a 5K, eventually.* She writes down the website on a small yellow college ruled pad of paper with her purple ball point pen.

The boys finish their bowls of Cheerios, get down from their chairs and go outside to play. Cooper grabs his basketball on the way out the door. Carson flies out the door and grabs his black BMX bike. Cooper shoots hoops while Carson is doing tricks on his bike.

Andrea cleans up the breakfast dishes and then sits down on the sectional couch with her laptop computer. She brings up the website of the 5K training program and sees that she can still sign up. Andrea proceeds to sign up for the 5K walking training program. Then she sends an email off to her ex-husband, Michael, letting him know that she signed up for the training program and will need him to watch the boys when she has training walks on Thursday evenings.

Putting her laptop on the table to the right of the couch, Andrea grabs her camera as she heads outside. She starts taking pictures of Carson on his bike doing tricks and Cooper shooting hoops.

Carson is riding around doing some bunny hops and going up and down on the ramps he has set up on the one side of the driveway.

Cooper is practicing his free throw shots. He's doing pretty good for a 5-year-old. Then he starts dribbling up and down the driveway in front of the garage of the townhouse.

Andrea sits down on the front porch continuing to take pictures of the boys while enjoying the heat of the sunshine. After taking quite a few pictures Andrea puts her camera down on the porch and walks over to join Cooper with his basketball. They have fun going back and forth trying to make shots while the other one blocks.

After playing outside for a few hours, they all head inside. The boys kick off their shoes on the mat by the front door, run upstairs to their bathroom, and get all washed up Andrea goes in the kitchen, washes her hands in the sink and gets the ingredients out of the refrigerator to make grilled cheese sandwiches for lunch.

Carson pops into the kitchen and asks, "Can I help?"

"Of course!" replies Andrea and she hands him the bread. "Lay out the bread on the cutting board." Carson places the slices of bread in a single layer on the cutting board.

Andrea is buttering the bread slices and Cooper comes sliding on the tile into the kitchen and says, "I want to help too!"

She hands him the slices of cheese and says to him "you get to put the cheese on all the bread slices that are buttered."

So, Cooper puts cheese slices on the bread slices that Andrea has buttered. Andrea then puts together the sandwiches and grills them on the stove. While the sandwiches are cooking Carson gets the plates out of the cupboard and Cooper brings the potato chips out and they set the table. The sandwiches get done and they all sit down to eat lunch.

While having lunch Andrea says to the boys, "I am going to do a training program and you boys will be with your dad while I am out training with my group. However, when I have homework walks you boys can go with me."

The boys get big smiles on their faces about the homework walks and say, "can we go now?"

Andrea explains, "It will be soon, but not yet."

They finish up their lunches, put all the dishes away and head back outside to play. This time Cooper grabs his bike and rides up and down the driveway. Carson once again practices his bunny hops and riding up and down the ramps. Andrea gets down next to her garden area and pulls out the weeds.

Andrea thinks to herself, *this nice garden area will have some great strawberries this summer that I'll be able to add to salads and smoothies.*

Andrea takes a break by sitting on the porch while the sun is getting a little bit lower in the sky. The boys are loving their bikes. Andrea says to herself, *I will go get my bike out and we can go for a bike ride.*

She then says to the boys "hey, let's all go for a bike ride" and the boys excitedly yell "YEAH!"

After closing up the townhouse they head down the sidewalk towards the bike trail. Andrea follows behind the boys so that she can keep an eye on them.

Andrea instills in the boys, "While on the sidewalk and trail you boys need to stay single file on the right side of the trail and to let people know when you come up behind them. We will go out for a little bit and then turn around and head back home."

"Alright boys let's turn around and head for home," she says. Carson and Cooper race back home. Carson wins by a tire. Both boys are very excited. Andrea gets there and opens the garage door so the boys can put their bikes in the garage along with the bike ramps. Then it's already time to get ready for dinner.

The boys go inside and get all washed up for dinner. Andrea heads into the kitchen and gets out the ingredients for dinner, which are salmon, carrots and rice. She thinks to herself I am looking forward to adding walking to my routine and slowly changing my diet for the better.

Andrea starts up the rice cooker with some sweet-smelling jasmine rice, slices up the carrots, putting the carrots in the cast iron skillet that is sprayed with an oil and finally puts the salmon in the cast iron skillet. She sprinkles the carrots and salmon with a lemon pepper seasoning and puts a lid on the skillet.

While waiting for the salmon, carrots and rice to cook Andrea sets the table and calls to the boys, "boys come to the table for dinner!" They sit down at the table and turn on the television, of course to watch Scooby Doo.

The rice cooker goes off. Andrea walks to the kitchen and plates up dinner for her and the boys bringing it into the dining room. Dinner is a big hit, as the boys ate everything on their plates. The boys take their dishes into the kitchen and put them in the dishwasher.

After dinner the boys head up to their rooms and sit at their desks to work on homework. Andrea cleans up the kitchen and then heads upstairs to help the boys with their homework. Once homework is complete the boys take a bath and get ready for bed.

It's been a busy day and both Carson and Cooper are really tired. They get in bed with no problems and go right to sleep. Andrea changes into her pajamas and sits down in the living room to relax and watch the Hallmark Channel.

Chapter 2: Getting Ready for Training

Two weeks later Andrea receives an email from the training program that tells her how to get ready for the training. The email includes where the best places are to get what she needs and what discounts she'll get at the various stores for being in the training program. Andrea prints out the email so that she can check off everything as she gets it all done.

She hollers upstairs to the boys, "Let's go shopping!"

Cooper and Carson come bounding down the stairs with their jackets on and run over to get their shoes on. They all get into Andrea's red F-350 crew cab truck and head into town.

They go to Bauman's Running and Walking Shop, where Adam greets them at the door. The boys go and sit with their tablets on the big red comfy couches.

Adam asks, "What are you looking for?"

Andrea replies, "I am starting the 5K walking training program."

"Congratulations on starting a great program," he replies.

Adam explains "We have a variety of shoes and I will need to see how you walk to determine which style will help you the best."

She then proceeds to take her shoes off so that Adam can see how her foot hits the ground when she walks away from him and towards him.

"Your foot overpronates. So, what that means is that your foot tolls inward too far when you walk. We have shoes that will help you with that. They are the stability shoes. Let's get your shoe size and then I'll grab a bunch of shoes from the back for you to try on," he says. Next Adam has her stand in the shoe sizer to make sure that he gets the right size.

Adam explains, "Now your feet will swell when you walk, so you are going to want to go up a half size from what it says right now because you haven't been out walking."

He then goes into the back room as Andrea takes a seat on the bench next to the boys. She leans over to see what the boys are watching on the tablets. Of course, they are watching Scooby Doo and have headphones on so they don't disturb anyone with the sound. Andrea sits back up and looks around the store at all the shoes on two of the walls and the large assortment of clothing on the racks.

Adam appears from the back room a short time later with six boxes of shoes stacked on top of each other. They are all different brands. He has them in her size to see how each one fits her foot and which one will be most comfortable. He sets them down on the floor and opens the first box explaining to her what that particular shoe is good for and how it will help her. He does this for all six pairs of shoes and he takes note of what she likes and dislikes about each shoe. After going through the six pairs of shoes and seeing how they all fit she finally decides on one pair of shoes.

Next up is getting socks that will work with the shoes and not against them. There are a few different brands on the market. Adam goes through the brands and what his recommendation is for a beginning walker. Andrea decides to get a few pair.

Her next question to Adam is "What do I do about clothing? How do I know what to wear and when?"

Adam explains to her "You should dress for 20 degrees warmer than what the thermometer says it is. If it says 50, dress for 70. You may be cold to start, but you will quickly warm up and be glad you dressed appropriately."

They have quite a few outfits for Andrea to mix and match. She has fun trying on various outfits to see how they actually feel. Some looked better on the hanger and she figures they may look better after she loses a few pounds or at least tones up. She decides on a couple outfits.

Adam then shows her the section where all the area races have their fliers at. He says, "these are free for the taking and with this training program the entry is included for the race. I am sure that once you are done with this one you will want to do more races and keep up the exercise regimen. Plus, the running & walking community is a great one and you will make lots of friends," Adam tells her.

He also shows her the area where she can get all kinds of other gear for walking. This area has a variety of water bottles, energy gels, stickers, magnets, fitness watches and sunglasses. Adam says, "You won't need to worry about these with just starting out, but they will come in handy as you progress after the 5K."

While checking out with her new walking gear a couple ladies enter the store. Adam says to Andrea, "These ladies are Vickie and Angela. Angela is one of the walking group trainers for your training program." He then says to Angela and Vickie, "This is Andrea and she has signed up for the 5K walking program."

Andrea is very excited to meet some ladies that are in the walking program. Angela explains, "The training program will help you successfully finish the race. You will be in a group of about eight participants. The groups vary in size according to ability. Included in your registration are weekly walks with the group, a training program t-shirt and cinch sack, discounts at various places including here, vouchers for two races in addition to the Oakland 5K, and 5 free visits to Fitness For Life gym. You are going to have a lot of fun, meet some great people and accomplish a 5K. We look forward to seeing you there."

Then the boys get up from the couch and come over by their mom. Andrea says to Angela and Vickie, "these are my boys, Carson and Cooper. Say Hi boys." "Hi," they both reply.

Andrea and the boys leave the store and head for home. When they get home Andrea parks in the garage and the boys grab her bags and head into townhouse. Upon entering the townhouse they kick off their shoes by the door. Then they take the bags into her room and lay them on her bed for her.

Andrea follows behind them and when she gets to her room she says to them, "You can stay if you want."

Carson and Cooper decide to head downstairs to watch some more Scooby Doo instead. Andrea then dumps out the bags on her bed. She admires her new outfits, cutting off the tags and placing them in a nicely cleared space in her dresser drawer. She is so excited to have her new shoes that she takes out a pair of new socks, puts them on and then puts on her new shoes. Andrea then heads downstairs and walks around the townhouse with her new shoes on for the rest of the evening.

Chapter 3: The First Evening

Finally, the first evening of training has arrived. Andrea yells upstairs to the boys "time to go!" The boys come bounding down the stairs and run over to get their coats and shoes on. Andrea picks up her gym bag and they all head to the garage, get in the truck and drive over to their dad's.

Carson says, "I can't wait to get to dad's!"

"Me, too!" adds Cooper.

Andrea drops off the boys with her ex, Michael, and then heads to Lutheran High's gym.

It's a pretty smooth drive as traffic moves without any problems and she arrives in the parking lot and finds a spot. Andrea gets out of her truck and heads in to the gym. There are a lot of people there already. She gets in the gym and follows the signs to the table where you check in at.

The gal at the table greets her, "My name is Anne."

Andrea says, "I am Andrea Walker."

Anne checks her name off the list, hands her a bag of goodies and says, "at the next table you will get your t-shirt."

When she gets to the next table the guy says, "Hi! I am Jim. What's your name?"

"I am Andrea Walker," she replies.

He then checks her name on the list and gets her a t-shirt. He informs her, "You can walk around the vendor tables until it's time to get started."

Andrea walks over to the vendor area. The first table that she stops at is a table with headbands. The gal at the headband table says, "Hi! I am Mary. Let me know if you need any assistance." Mary has all kinds of headbands with various fun phrases about running and walking. Andrea buys a purple one that says "I don't sweat, I sparkle."

She continues on to the next table where a local race is being promoted and she puts a flier in her bag. She continues to make her way looking at the tables from a distance. There's one from a chiropractic office, a running store, and a gal with a protein drink. Andrea decides to go over to the bleachers and sit down until the next part of the program starts.

A few minutes later Anne steps up to the microphone located in front of the bleachers at the microphone and says, "Welcome to the Oakland Training Program! I am so glad that everyone could make it and for those that haven't made it to their seats yet, please make your way there quickly. We are going to get started in a couple minutes, and give people a chance to get to their seats."

Vickie and Kim walk up and Vickie says, "Hi Andrea! This is Kim. Kim, I met Andrea at Bauman's Running and Walking Shop. She is in the 5K walking program."

"Hi Andrea! Glad to have you be part of the program," Kim says. "Denese will be joining us shortly."

Andrea replies, "Nice to meet you Kim. I am looking forward to walking."

Denese walks up, "Hi, I am Denese."

"Hi Denese, I am Andrea. Glad to meet you," Andrea replies.

Five minutes later Anne gets back to the microphone and says, "Welcome to the Oakland Training Program! We are going to get started. I'd like to welcome all of our first-time participants. Would all of our first-time participants please stand up!" Andrea stands up along with a bunch of others. "Welcome! Congratulations on joining us! You can have a seat.

What we are going to do tonight is head out to the track and have everyone walk the track for one lap. Please do this at a pace you are comfortable with. You do NOT want to go too fast. We are determining which group to put you in and it's better to be in a slower group than a group that is too fast for you. At the end of your lap you will receive a popsicle stick with a number on it. You will bring that stick back to the table that is right inside the door. Give them the stick, tell them whether you are walking or running and your name. This will put you into groups. We will then meet back here in the bleachers when everyone is done. So, go ahead and head out to the track."

Andrea, Vickie, Kim and Denese all head to the track together. They are joined by a bunch of other walkers and runners on the track. The gentleman that is already at the track instructs them, "All right everyone, gather behind the line. I need one group of eight on the track at the line and then when that group is done another group of 8 will go until we are all done."

He then counts down and has them head off on the track. Andrea thinks to herself *I like this. Walking feels good, these people are so nice and the sun is shining!*

It didn't take long, and they found themselves at the finish line grabbing the popsicle sticks. They then leave the track and head back to the gym to turn in their popsicle sticks. There were two lines, one for runners and one for walkers. They all lined up in the walker line, gave them their popsicle stick, confirmed they were walkers and gave their name. Once all of them are done with that they walk over to the bleachers where they sit down and continue to chat while everyone files in from the track.

Anne walks up to the microphone again and says, "Welcome back everyone! We will take a few more minutes while the groups get divided up amongst our leaders and then you will get with your group and go out for a short walk." She walks over to the table and grabs the group sheets that are ready and walks back over to the microphone.

"Ok, I have some of the group sheets already available and we'll get those groups started off walking or running with your assigned group leader. Our first group is for group leader Angela Green. Angela, please come up here. Now I will call off the names of the group members. They can join Angela up here and then head out for their walk. Those trainees are Andrea Walker, Vickie Haus, Kim Gross, Karin Tallasman, Denese Wilcox, Doree Lakeland, and Sharon East. Come on down and join Angela! Happy walking!"

They all join Angela on the gym floor. Angela says, "let's go outside, we'll talk a bit and get walking." They all follow Angela outside. "Welcome! I am so glad to have you ladies as my group of trainees. We are going to start out slow so that we can figure out where everyone is at pace wise. Each week we will go at the pace of the slowest walker that evening. There will be evenings that everyone is at the back of the pack. This is normal. No one is at their best every single week. You will have "off" weeks and that's OK. The object of this training program is get you walking and finish the race. Let's walk over to my car and we can drop our bags in the back of my car so your hands are free while walking." Everyone walks over to Angela's 2009 black Chevrolet HHR and puts their bags in the back end. "Alright, let's get walking!" Angela says.

"Now the first thing we will cover is walking etiquette. We will walk 2 by 2. So, no more than 2 people wide. This will help us immensely on the trails. When a car comes up behind us the person at the back will shout out "Car Back." When a car comes towards us the person in front shouts out "Car Up." When we have another group that comes up behind us and is going to pass us the person in the back shouts out "runners or walkers back" and then the whole group moves into a single file line to allow the other group to pass by. If there is a bicycle that comes up behind us the person at the back also shouts "bike back" and if they know how many they shout "2 bikes back" if there are two bikes coming. Sometimes you will know and other times the bikes will come up very quickly and you will only have time to say "bikes back." No worries it's only a warning. The person in the front will shout "runners or walkers up" when a group is approaching. Our group will go into single file line and then it's always a great thing to give the passing group a high five. They will also shout "bike or bikes up" when there are oncoming bikes. We will get over to a single file line if the path is too narrow for the bikes to safely pass us. Another thing that the front person will shout out is if there is a problem with the path, such as hole in path or low branches or something similar. When we are on sidewalks this will be more common with uneven sidewalk. Does anyone have any questions?" Everyone shakes their head no.

"I will also give directions of which way we are going, such as left or right or straight across depending on what the direction will be. I will have the map printed out ahead of time and we can look at it before we head out next time. Also, expect a weekly email from me with where we will be meeting, possibly a map of what our next route will be, what our distance and time was the previous walk, what our homework is and who is responsible for snacks. When we get back to my car I have a list of weeks and everyone can sign up for a week that is good for them to bring a snack. Snacks that are typically brought are raisins, grapes, strawberries, oranges, fruit snacks, granola bars and such. Also, water is good for after our walk."

"Ok, we are almost back to the parking lot. We will head over to my car." They walk through the parking lot to Angela's car. "How was the pace for everyone?" Everyone replies that it was a good pace. Angela passes around the snack chart. Andrea picks week 4 to bring a snack. "OK, I will see everyone next week at 6:00 in the north parking lot of Oakland High School that faces University Dr." Everyone says "See you next week!"

Andrea grabs her bag and walks to her truck. Time to go get the boys from their dad's.

A few minutes later she pulls up in her ex's driveway. She goes up and rings the doorbell. Cooper runs to the door and opens it yelling

"MOM'S HERE!" Carson comes running, too, and they both get their coats and shoes on. Their dad gives them both a hug and kiss goodbye. The boys and Andrea go to the truck and drive home.

It was a busy evening. As soon as they get in the door to the townhouse they take their shoes off and the boys head upstairs to put on their pajamas. They brush their teeth and say good night.

Andrea sits down on the couch for a few minutes to relax in the silence for a thirty minutes and heads upstairs to go to sleep herself.

Chapter 4: Stretching Homework

It's Friday evening and the boys have left with their dad for the weekend. Andrea has the townhouse to herself and decides to do her homework for the training program. She goes to her goodie bag that she received at the training program the evening before. Andrea pulls out the training schedule. She finds that today's homework is stretching. Andrea thinks to herself that it is very doable.

Andrea goes upstairs to change into some comfortable clothes do to stretching exercises in. She decides on a pair of black running shorts and a purple tank top. Andrea walks back downstairs to the living room.

She grabs her stretching booklet that is with the training homework and lays it on the floor. She sits down on the carpeted floor and proceeds to read through the exercises. Andrea takes each exercise out and lays them out on the floor and starts doing her stretches.

The first exercise is a squat with a reach. So, Andrea stands up and places her feet wider than her shoulders and keeps her upper body tall. She proceeds to squat by sticking her butt back while keeping her upper body tall. When she gets to the bottom of her squat she reaches both her hands forward. Andrea continues to do these ten times in a row and then takes a brief break to get a drink of water from the glass she has sitting on the table. She then continues for a second set of ten squats and reaches.

After Andrea completes her squats she moves on to her second exercise that is the single leg shoulder press. She then stands on her right leg with the left foot a couple inches off the ground. Taking her left hand she makes a fist and presses her fist as high as she can. Her hip naturally is out a bit when she raises her left foot up and when she has her hand as high as she can press up her hip straightens out. She brings her arm down and puts her foot back on the floor. She repeats the exercise 12 times on each side.

For the next exercise, which is called rapid reaching, Andrea grabs a small stack of books. Andrea then stands on her right leg, bends at the hip and her upper body stays straight and falls forward. She proceeds to reach with her right hand to touch the books and then with her left, alternating between them. Andrea touches the books with each of her hands 12 times. She stands on her left foot and repeats the exercise.

Andrea takes a short break after the last exercise to grab a drink of water. She looks down at the stretches and sees that the next exercise which is warrior II. Andrea stands with her feet shoulder width apart and her toes pointed straight forward. She then turns her right foot to the right while turning her body to face the right. Andrea raises her arms out to her sides and then bends her right knee to have her knee over her foot. She checks to make sure she can still see her toes. As she presses her feet apart she gazes over her right middle finger. Andrea holds her position and takes four deep breaths. Andrea straightens her right leg and then turns her right foot and body back forward. Then she repeats the exercise with the left foot.

Andrea thinks to herself, *I can't believe I am doing these exercises.* Her next exercise is the walker's arms. Andrea stands with her right foot forward, sucks in her stomach, and bends her arms at the elbow to a 90-degree angle. She moves her arms alternately forward and backward. Andrea does this for 20 forward movements for each arm and then switches to her left foot, and repeats the arm exercise on this foot forward.

When she completes the walker's arms she looks down at her exercises and sees that she is on exercise six which is the plank. Andrea thinks to herself that it should be interesting to see how well this goes. She puts down the stretching booklet and then gets down on the floor. Andrea proceeds to get down on her hands while straightening her legs out and is on her toes. She gets her back flat keeping in angle with her straight legs. She holds this position slowly counting to 15. She puts her knees down for a few second break and then straightens her legs again. This time she held the position slowly counting to 20. Andrea takes another few second break and takes the position one last time and holds it slowly counting to 20.

Andrea then sits down after her planks. She thinks to herself, *I am very pleased with how well I have done for the first time.* While sitting down on the floor she looks over her stretching exercises that are laid out on the floor. Her next exercise is called super hero. This one looks really interesting as it requires some balancing. Andrea puts down the stretching booklet and moves to get on her hands and knees. She makes sure that her hands are directly below her shoulders and her knees are a hip width apart. Andrea then extends her right arm out front and her left leg behind her. She holds the position slowly counting to 20 and then switches to her left arm and right leg. Andrea does this for five times on each side.

She completes her super heroes and moves on to exercise number eight which is walking knee hugs. Andrea puts down the exercise booklet and then stands up nice and tall. She then walks forward with her right leg first and brings her left knee up hugging it to her chest. Andrea continues doing this alternating her knees and going forward one step at a time. She makes sure to keep her back nice and straight while she does this for ten knee hugs on each leg.

Andrea glances down to her exercises and the next exercise is the triangle. She stands with her feet a little bit wider than shoulder width apart and her toes pointed forward. Then brings her arms up to form a "T," turns her right foot to the right and then bends at the waist reaching her right hand down to her right foot and turns her head to look up to her left hand keeping her arms straight. Andrea takes five deep breaths and rises back up to form a "T" again. She repeats this to the left side.

Rising back up to a "T" after her left side and for the next exercise of revolving forward bend she bends at her waist to keep her upper body at a 90-degree angle and she reaches down with her hands on the floor. Next Andrea walks her hands over to her right foot and lifts her right hand up towards the ceiling and looks up to her hand. She holds it for 5 deep breaths and then lowers her hand and walks her hands to her left foot and lifts her left hand, looks up to her hand and holds the position for 5 deep breathes.

After she completes the left side of her revolving forward bend she stands back up and then gets down on her hands and knees with her shoulders over her hands and back straight to get into position for the downward dog exercise. She then curls her toes under while lifting her hips up and back as she straightens her legs. Andrea holds this position for five deep breaths. She moves back down to her knees on the floor.

Andrea gets up off the floor and takes a drink of water while looking down at the exercises to see that she is on her last stretching exercise of supine spinal twist. She reads the description and smiles thinking to herself that she is glad this is the last one and it is lying down. Andrea lays down on her back on the floor. She brings her arms out to a "T", brings her right knee up to a 90-degree angle and drops it to her left side. She then turns her head to look down her right arm to her fingertips. Andrea holds it for 5 deep breaths and brings her right knee back up and lays it down next to her left leg. She then repeats with her left leg.

When Andrea is done with her left leg and lays it back down she lays there for a few moments only enjoying her own thoughts of how well she did her first set of stretching exercises. After a few moments, she sits up, picks up the exercise pages, puts them in her booklet, finishes her water and walks out to the kitchen to get some more water.

She returns to the living room where her goodie bag for the training program is, picks up a pen that was in the bag and puts a smiley face on the training program calendar for today's stretches.

Smiling and thinking to herself, I love what all I have done so far. I will treat myself to a hot bath and a movie.

Chapter 5: Week 2

Michael comes up to the door and rings the doorbell. Carson comes running down the stairs with Cooper right behind him. They are very excited to see their dad. Carson opens the door and jumps on his dad. Michael puts him down on the floor and tells them, "get your shoes on we are going for dinner."

The boys yell up to their mom, "MOOOMMMM, dad's here, we're leaving!"

Andrea comes down from her room and tells them, "be good for your dad, I will see you when I get back from walking." She kisses them both on the forehead. Michael, Carson and Cooper all leave for dinner.

Andrea goes into the living room, puts her shoes on, grabs her walking bag and heads out the door. She gets into her truck and drives to Oakland High School.

A short drive later she arrives in the parking lot at Oakland High School and finds Angela's car. Angela is sitting in the back of her car with the hatch open listening to some country music. Andrea is early enough that she can get a parking spot right next to Angela. She parks her truck, picks up her walking bag, gets out of her truck and walks up to Angela.

"Hello!" says Angela.

"Hi" Andrea replies.

"So, what did you think of the homework?" inquires Angela.

Andrea responds, "I was really impressed that I could do the stretching exercises the first time through and that I got my walking in."

"I am glad to hear it. You can actually do those stretching exercises every day if you like. They will help with your walking." Says Angela.

Vickie walks up, "Hi ladies!"

"Hi!" both Andrea and Angela reply. "How did the homework go?" asks Angela.

"Really well." Responds Vickie.

Kim, Denese and Doree all walk up together.

"Hi!" Angela says.

They all reply, "Hi!"

"Did we all do our homework?" inquires Angela.

"Yes!" they all responded in unison.

Sharon drives by them with the window rolled down, "be right there" she says and continues along to find her parking spot. After parking Sharon comes over and joins the rest of the group.

Karin walks up at the same time Sharon does. Angela asks them, "did you ladies do your homework?"

They both answer, "yes."

"Ok, now that we are all here," Angela talks with them. "We are going to be going out for our 20-minute walk. We'll do 10 minutes across University and then back. Tonight's treat was brought by Vickie." "Ready?"

"Ready!" responded everyone.

"As a reminder, we need to stay in 2 by 2 format walking on these sidewalks. The person in back will watch out for other groups and bikers coming up behind us. The person in front will do the same for oncoming groups and bikers." Angela reminds the group.

"This evening we are going to be doing interval training. We will walk a faster pace for 1 minute and then a 30 second slower pace. This will enable to go further and faster in the end. When you are walking your faster pace keep your arms at a 90-degree angle and pump them. Thus, when we go to do our faster pace I will shout Arms Up! When we switch to the slower pace we will put our arms down and I will shout Arms Down! I have the intervals on my watch. You will feel your muscles being sore in a few days. Make sure to do your stretches. I know they are on the schedule for certain days, but you can do them every day if you like. Remember to focus on the form and not the speed." Angela informs them. "Let's go! Arms up!" she shouts as she starts them out walking.

They start out on the sidewalk next to the parking lot and head north for a few yards or so to the sidewalk that goes along University. University is a very busy road and thus very noisy. So, Angela has to talk a bit louder to make sure that everyone hears her. "Arms down!" she shouts and then 30 seconds later "arms up!" This continues throughout their walk.

Angela is at the front of the group. The ladies are all talking amongst themselves.

"How are your boys?" Angela asks Andrea.

"They are great. I dropped them off at their dad's on my way here. I told them about the homework I will have and they both got big smiles and wanted to go out walking right away. Walking with the boys this spring and summer and getting my homework completed, too, will be fun."

"Awesome. Glad to hear they are supportive. How is their dad with your training?"

"He is pretty supportive. I just emailed him about the training and he will work with me. He does on a regular basis anyways. We get along much better apart then we did together. So, training will be pretty easy in that aspect. He's already said that he'll have the boys at the finish line for me."

"That's great. It's nice to see exes getting along so well and working together."

"Yes, it makes things much easier for all of us."

"Our turn around point is coming up shortly and we'll head back."

"I can't believe we are already to our turn around point. It seems like we just started. It certainly is easier walking with a group then by yourself."

"Yes, it is. I love doing the training groups much better than training by myself. Although there are times when I want to think things out and walking by myself works much better."

Next Angela yells to everyone, "we will be turning around here, so everyone behind me again." A few moments after they turn around another group is coming towards them. "Runners up! Everyone single file!" Angela shouts to her group. As the runners go by Angela and her group they give the other group high five's and say, "great job."

After the runners go by the group falls back into 2 by 2 formation. They arrive back at the cars a few minutes later. Kim goes over to her car, pops open the trunk and gets out a cooler full of goodies. She brings it over to Angela's car and puts it in the open hatch area that Angela had opened. Kim says, "we have green seedless grapes and sliced strawberries in baggies and bottles of water."

"Thank you, Kim, for bringing the treats this evening and next week is Vickie's turn," says Angela. "Let's go over how we did tonight. We did a 1 minute faster walk with a 30 second slower walk. How does that work for everyone?" she asks.

"Worked for me" says Karin.

"Yeah" agrees the rest of the ladies.

"Ok, so next week we will keep the same intervals. We will meet downtown at the library parking lot that is on the west end of the parking lot or the one closest to Main Street." Angela informs them. "See you next week!"

They finish their goodies and disperse to their vehicles. Andrea gets into her truck, puts her water bottle into the cup holder and backs out of her parking space. She leaves the parking lot and heads for home, as Michael is taking the boys back home after they have dinner.

It's a short drive and she's already home. She pulls into her garage, parks the truck, picks up her stuff, gets out of the truck and goes inside. "Boys, I am home!" Andrea shouts as she opens the door.

"YEAH!!!!" yell the boys as they come running to her from the living room.

"We got to go to The Buffet for dinner! Then we watched Scooby Doo!!" the boys tell her.

"Yes, they also got some reading homework done." Michael lets her know. Andrea nods her head in acknowledgment.

"Well, I will head for home now." Michael says.

"Bye daddy!" both the boys tell him and give him a big hug goodbye. "We love you!" they shout as Michael leaves.

"I love you guys too." Michael replies as he goes out the door.

"Time for bed boys." Andrea tells them.

They run up the stairs and into their bedroom. Opening their dressers, they get their pajamas out and change into them. Once they are changed they jump into their beds. A few minutes later Andrea goes up the stairs and into the boys' bedroom.

"Great job getting ready for bed. Do you have a book ready to read?" she asks them.

"YES!" they both excitedly reply and Cooper hands her a book.

Andrea reads them their book, "the end. Time to sleep now." She pulls their covers up, shuts out the light, and says, "Good night boys, love you."

"Love you mom," they say back.

Angela walks into her room and gets ready for bed. She picks up her walking booklet that has her schedule and stretching exercises in it. Andrea sits down and looks over her schedule.

She says to herself, *I'll start doing these exercises every day starting tomorrow.* Andrea puts the booklet down on her night stand, lays down, pulls the covers up, and goes to sleep.

Chapter 6: Walking Homework

It's a beautiful warm, sunny Saturday morning and Andrea is just waking up to the sun shining through the window blinds into her upstairs room. The townhouse is still quiet, as the boys haven't woke up yet.

Andrea thinks to herself, *today's homework is a 15-minute walk. Time to get up and get motivated. Do I eat first? Do I go for my walk first? What should I wear? Gotta get the boys up and moving with me.*

After lying in bed a few more minutes she finally gets up and takes a shower and gets ready to go for her walk. She picks out her black running shorts and purple tank top and lays them on her bed while she showers.

Her hot and steamy shower is done. Andrea gets dressed for her walk and she wakes up the boys. "Boys, time to get up! We're going out for a walk!" she says to the boys.

Cooper wakes up and takes a long stretch while still in bed; opening his eyes he says, "can I ride my bike?"

Andrea responds to him with "of course you can."

Carson peeks his eyes open and in a very groggy voice say, "do I have to get up?"

"Yes" she tells him. "You can ride your bike too."

Cooper bounces out of bed, gets his clothes changed and runs downstairs to the kitchen. Carson slowly sits up, then slowly puts his feet on the floor and very slowly gets dressed. He then sits on his butt and slides down the stairs.

In the kitchen, Andrea is setting the table for the boys to eat some cereal. For herself she mixes up her protein smoothie of Phyzix MD

Daily Pro - Dutch Chocolate Vegan, coconut milk, banana, natural unsweetened cocoa and extra crunchy peanut butter. The boys sit down at the table and eat their cereal. Andrea has her protein smoothie and is cleaning the kitchen up so that when the boys are done with their cereal they can get moving.

The boys put their cereal bowls and spoons in the dishwasher and go put their shoes on. Andrea puts her shoes on and takes her protein smoothie with her as they all go into the garage to get the boys' bikes. She opens the door for the boys, they each go out the door and wait in the driveway while she locks the door.

Andrea turns on her fitness watch to track her route, pace and time during her walk. They start out on the sidewalk going to the right. The boys go ahead of her.

"Not too far ahead boys!" she shouts.

The boys stop to let her catch up. They get to a corner and she checks her watch. They have been walking for 5 minutes. She sees a turnaround point up ahead to the right and tells the boys, "you guys can go to that fire hydrant and wait for me."

They speed on ahead of her. Andrea's watch is doing the 1-minute fast walk, 30 second slower walk intervals.

The boys get to the fire hydrant and stop. Finally, Andrea gets there, and she says, "time to turn around and head back for home."

They race to the corner, where Carson wins the race. "I won!" yells Carson. They wait patiently for Andrea to catch up.

She finally gets to the corner and tells the boys "you can ride home now." The boys race home. Cooper wins this time.

"Ha! I won!!!" yells Cooper. Cooper lays his bike down and picks up a basketball he had left outside and starts shooting hoops.

Carson rides back and forth in the driveway waiting for Andrea to make it home.

Andrea gets to the driveway and stops her fitness watch walk. She thinks to herself, *I am pleased with my walking time and that I got up and went out walking.*

Andrea unlocks the garage door and then the house door, goes inside, sets down her empty bottle of her protein smoothie, takes a bottle of Phyzix MD Energy Stix Natural Mixed Berry out of the fridge that she had premixed, grabs her tablet and goes out the front door to sit down on the front porch.

The boys are playing, and Andrea gets to read her e-book. As she sits on the front porch she looks up from her book and thinks to herself *I am grateful that the boys are exercising and having fun.* So, she sits her tablet down and joins Cooper playing basketball.

Carson puts his bike down and says "I'm hungry! Is it time for lunch?"

Andrea checks her fitness watch and says, "Yes, it is. Let's go inside for some lunch." They put up their things, go in through the garage and into the house.

Andrea goes into the kitchen and prepares the boys' lunch. Cooper gets a strawberry jelly sandwich and Carson gets a peanut butter sandwich. Andrea fixes herself an apple cinnamon jelly and extra crunchy peanut butter sandwich. They eat at the kitchen table sharing a bag of baked potato chips and tray of green seedless grapes.

After they finish eating Andrea cleans up the kitchen and the boys go into the living room to watch some tv. Once the kitchen is all cleaned up she goes into the living room and turns off the tv.

"Ok boys let's do some exercises."

"Awe mom!!! We want to watch tv" the boys reply.

After a few exercises from her booklet, "let's stand up and do some jumping jacks." The boys get up and do some jumping jacks with her.

"Now let's fly like superheroes" and they follow her lead of lying on their stomach and pretending to fly.

"Let's jump like a frog!" The boys respond with "ribbit, ribbit."

"Alright, now walk like a duck." The boys are now quacking.

"Ok, now you can watch some tv. I'll continue my exercises."

"Yeah!" they both reply.

Carson turns on the tv and turns it immediately to Scooby Doo.

Andrea completes her exercises and sits down on the couch. She grabs her laptop and catches up on Facebook, Instagram, Twitter and email.

Looking at the time on her laptop, Andrea sees that it's almost time for dinner. "Hey boys, what do you want for dinner?"

"Pizza!" they both exclaimed.

"Ok, I'll prepare it while you guys watch tv."

She goes out to the kitchen, gets the cheese and pepperoni out of the refrigerator, the pizza sauce out of the pantry, and the English muffins out of the bread box.

Opening the oven to make sure nothing is in there, she thinks to herself, *with boys, you never know what you might find. Nope, nothing in the oven.* Andrea turns it on to 375 degrees, grabs a cookie sheet, sprays it with non-stick spray, pries apart the English muffins and lays them on the cookie sheet.

Next up is spreading the pizza sauce on all of the English muffins along with sprinkling the shredded pizza cheese very liberally on the pizza sauce. Carson doesn't like pepperoni, so his pizzas are done. Cooper likes pepperoni and so does Andrea, so those get 6 pepperonis each on them and then more pizza cheese on top of the pepperonis. The oven is preheated now, so in the pizzas go and she turns the light on so that she can watch them get done.

"Boys! Pizzas are in the oven, get washed up and sit down at the dining room table," she yells to them.

They immediately get up and go to the bathroom to wash their hands and then sit down at the dining room table.

Checking the pizzas, they look done, as the cheese is all melted. Taking an oven mitt, she takes them out of the oven and sets them on the stove top.

Grabbing plates out of the cupboard above she puts four muffins on each plate, of course Carson's are the ones with only cheese. Andrea takes the boys' plates out to the dining room, gets them a glass of Crystal Light Wild Strawberry Energy with ice and then brings her own plate and drink to the table.

"These are YUMMMM…..MMMMMYYYY," says Carson.

"I like them too!" chimes in Cooper.

"Glad you both like them. They are quick and easy to make for you guys."

"How about after dinner you guys go outside and play?" she says to the boys.

"Yeah!" both boys answered.

The boys finish their pizzas, take their plates out to the kitchen and put them in the dishwasher. They come back out to the dining room table to get their glasses and put those in the dishwasher too.

Andrea finishes her pizzas and takes her plate and glass out to the kitchen and puts them in the dishwasher as well.

They all go outside. Carson rides his bike and does some bunny hops and rides up and down the ramps. Cooper shoots hoops and dribbles around the driveway. Andrea gets his Dribble Stick out and he dribbles around the Dribble Stick.

She thinks to herself, *it is great to watch the boys do what they enjoy doing.* The sun is starting to set just over the trees. Andrea says to the boys, "time to go in and get ready for bed."

"Ok," they both answer. Carson puts his bike away and Cooper puts his basketball and Dribble Stick away. They go in the house through the garage and then upstairs to get ready for bed.

Andrea goes in the front door and goes upstairs to the boys' room. "Good night," she tells them and gives them a hug and kiss on the forehead.

"Good night," they both reply.

She goes downstairs, sits down on the couch, reclines back and relaxes while watching her favorite channel, the Hallmark Channel.

Chapter 7: Week 3

Andrea changes into her walking clothes and goes downstairs. "Boys, time to get your shoes on to go to your dad's"

"YEAH!" they shout and run to put on their shoes.

They go out and get into Andrea's truck and off to their dad's they go. Along the way the boys are singing with the songs on the radio, one of their favorites is *I Play Chicken with The Train* by Cowboy Troy. It's a short ride and they arrive at their dad's. As soon as Andrea parks the truck, the boys get out of the truck and run up to the door. They stand there banging on the front door, yelling "DAD!" until Michael comes to the front door and opens it.

Carson and Cooper wave good bye and yell, "BYE MOM!"

Time to get moving on to training, Andrea backs out of the driveway and drives over to the Oakland library parking lot. Traffic is picking up in downtown Oakland, so the drive is a bit slower and more patience is required. She finds a nice parking spot under a tree and no one on one side of her. Andrea parks her truck, grabs her walking bag, gets out and walks over to Angela's car where Vickie, Karin, Sharon and Doree are already waiting.

"Hi!" Andrea says when she walks up.

"Hi!" they reply.

"Has everyone been doing their homework?" Angela asks.

"Yes," everyone replies.

"I have found it pretty easy to get out and exercise with my boys and they have enjoyed it as well," Andrea says.

"I am sure they do like it. Most kids will enjoy exercising, especially if it is in the form of playing. The more fun it is, the easier it is to get them to participate," Angela adds.

Shortly Kim and Denese walk up and join the group. Angela greets them, "welcome ladies! We are going to head out on the trail and go north for about 13 minutes and turn around and come back. We should get to Tienken Rd where we will turn around. If we need a few extra minutes we will cut through the park. We will head out 2 by 2 on the path. Ready ladies?"

"Ready!" everyone replied.

The ladies head out on the path 2 by 2 going under the main road where the creek is flowing over the scattered rocks. The sound is quite loud as it echoes in the tunnel. Some of the path is wet from the splashing of the water. When they get to the end of tunnel they can smell the hot dogs cooking from the restaurant that is next to the trail. There is an incline coming up from the tunnel as they go onto the wooded trail.

As they get onto the wooded trail there's a running group coming towards them. "Runners up! Single file!" yelled Andrea.

Everyone moves to a single file line and then gives high fives and says, "Good job" "Keep it up" "Looking good." The group moves past them and they go back to 2 by 2.

The wooded trail goes alongside a park and they can hear a band playing Rockin' Robin in the amphitheater. The ladies do a little dance along the trail and then go back to walking in the intervals of 1 minute fast walk or "arms up" and 30 seconds of slow walk or "arms down."

On their way along the trail they come into a clearing on the right. They see a fence that is for a day-care and in the fence is an American Flag made with red, white and blue plastic drinking cups. Next there is a ball field in the short distance where kids are playing.

Someone must have done something good as the crowd is cheering and clapping.

They come across the first intersection where Angela stops the group to make sure that traffic is stopping, once traffic stops she goes into the middle of the intersection and stops to make sure that all of her trainees are safely on the other side. She then joins them, and they continue along the trail.

Up ahead on the trail a deer stands in the middle of the trail looking towards the group. Andrea and Vickie are at the front of the group and they slow their pace. Vickie turns to Andrea, whispers "deer" and points at the deer. Andrea nods her head.

Vickie turns around to Kim and Denese, whispers "deer" and points at the deer. They both nod.

Kim turns around to Karin and Doree, whispers "deer" and points at the deer. They both nod.

Doree turns around to Sharon and Angela, whispers "deer" and points at the deer. They both nod.

They all quietly and slowly continue toward the deer. The deer stays still for a while and then casually walks off the trail to the west. The ladies return to their previous pace and continue along the trail to the next intersection of Tienken Rd where they turn around and head back.

This time when they get to the next intersection Andrea waits for traffic to clear and then she walks out into the middle of the intersection to make sure everyone gets across and then joins Angela at the back of the group.

Once they all get across they take the trail that goes through the park along the creek. There are a dozen ducks that are quacking and splashing along the creek beside them.

They get closer to the amphitheater and they can hear the music again, this time the band is playing Rock Around the Clock. At the end of the park they have to return to the trail where they go down the hill and through the tunnel next to the creek and under the road. The ladies finish up their walk right next to Angela's car.

Vickie gets the snacks out of her vehicle. "I brought watermelon slices and water."

Angela informs her group, "Great walk ladies! How awesome to see the deer and the ducks along our walk and hear some great music. Next week we will meet at Oakland High School North on Tienken Rd. Also, Andrea has next week's snacks. See everyone next week!"

The ladies all say, "good-bye," then they all go to their vehicles.

Andrea gets into her truck and heads for home. She has a text message that says Michael took the boys home. She has a nice short drive home, parks her truck in the garage and goes inside. "Carson! Cooper! I am home!" Andrea shouts as she enters the townhouse.

The boys come running to greet her and give her hugs. "Mom!" they both shout. They are already in their pajamas.

Michael says to the boys, "time for me to go, give me a hug." The boys go over and give him a hug.

"Good night Carson," he says and kisses him on the forehead.

"Good night dad."

"Good night Cooper," he says and kisses him on the forehead.

"Good night dad."

He gives them both another hug and then leaves for home.

"Time for bed boys!" Andrea tells Cooper and Carson. The boys run upstairs, go into the bathroom, brush their teeth, go into their room and jump into bed.

Andrea goes upstairs and tucks them in bed with kisses on their foreheads. She then goes into her room, gets her pajamas on, and climbs into bed.

The moon light is peeking in her room through the blinds, she picks up her phone and opens the music app to select her relaxation play list. Laying her phone back on the nightstand she picks up her tablet and opens the eBook that she has been reading.

Her mind drifts away to the evening walk, *I never thought I'd be in a walking group, let alone doing so well. What great friends I have made, and I feel great. It's just week three and so much more to come.*

Setting her tablet down on the nightstand, she settles down into her blankets and goes off to sleep.

Chapter 8: Track Workout and Beyond

The sun is coming up in the east, peeking over the tree tops, painting the sky bright blue with no clouds in sight. In the tree outside of Andrea's window the birds are chirping, and the squirrels are chattering. Across her room is an essential oil diffuser emitting a comforting blend of Peppermint, Eucalyptus, Cypress, Lemon and Elemi. Andrea lays in her bed looking out the window and listening to all of the sounds of the morning. The boys have not yet woken up. *Time to get up*, she thinks to herself putting on her robe and opening her bedroom door.

She walks over to the boys' bedroom and opens the door. Both are still asleep, and she goes downstairs to the kitchen.

Andrea makes herself a large cup of hot cocoa with mini marshmallows. She lets it sit on the counter while the mini marshmallows melt across the top of the mug.

This morning's breakfast is going to be scrambled eggs mixed with ham and mushrooms. First Andrea chops up the mushrooms and puts them in a cast iron skillet along with some butter and minced garlic. She lets those cook up while stirring them periodically to keep them from burning. In between stirring Andrea dices up the ham, and adds the ham to mushrooms, mixing them all together.

Suddenly Carson comes running down the stairs and into the kitchen, "mom, are we having ham for breakfast?!" he excitedly questions as he slides across the kitchen floor towards the stove to look into the skillet.

"Yes, Carson, we are having scrambled eggs with ham and mushrooms," Andrea replies.

They hear Cooper bounding down the stairs and into the kitchen, "do I smell ham?" Cooper exclaims.

"Yes, Cooper, you smell ham. We are having scrambled eggs with ham and mushrooms," Andrea answers him.

"Ok boys wash up and get dressed, after breakfast we are going over to the track," she tells them.

"Yeah!" they reply and dash out of the kitchen and up the stairs to their room.

Meanwhile, Andrea mixes together eggs, coconut milk, and Canadian steak seasoning. She pours the egg mixture into the ham and mushrooms. The boys hurriedly come down the stairs and into the kitchen and sit down in their seats. Andrea finishes up the scrambled eggs, prepares the boys' plates and takes them their eggs. She makes her own plate and sits down, eating breakfast with her boys.

Carson and Cooper are all done with their breakfast. They put their plates in the dishwasher, get their shoes on and go into the garage to take out their bikes. Andrea cleans up the kitchen, goes upstairs to get her walking clothes on, comes back downstairs and out into the garage to get the boys.

Andrea opens the side door of the garage, the boys ride their bikes outside, she steps out into the bright warm sun and she locks the door behind them.

Carson leads on his bike, closely followed by Cooper.

Andrea says to the boys, "stop at the corner."

She catches up to them at the corner. They all wait for the light to change and walk across together. The school track is a quarter mile from the corner. Carson leads them to the entrance of the school parking lot and stops to wait for Cooper and Andrea to catch up to him. They catch up and Cooper and Carson race to the track. Andrea meets up with them at the entrance to the track.

"Alright boys, you guys stay to the outside of the track," says Andrea to the boys as they head out onto the track on their bikes.

For the long stretch of the track she goes as fast as she can walk and reaches the first curve at the end and switches into walking knee hugs along the curve. When she reaches the next curve, she walks as fast as she can again through the straight away section. Andrea repeats her walking knee hugs along the curved section of the track. She gets to the straight away section and catches up to the boys. They look behind them and see her and take off down the track again. Andrea does her track workout for two more laps. Carson and Cooper are laughing and racing around the track on their bikes.

As she finishes up her last walking knee hug interval, Andrea walks over to the entrance to the track and yells out to the boys, "Hey boys! Time to go home!"

They race over to Andrea. "Let's go!"

Carson races ahead to the track gate, Cooper follows close behind him. When she gets to the gate the boys race to through the parking lot and to the sidewalk where they stop to wait for her. Andrea catches up to them.

She reminds them, "wait for me at the traffic light."

Cooper takes off in front this time with Carson following a few yards behind him. They get to the traffic light and stop and wait for Andrea to catch up. She gets to the traffic light, it changes and they all cross together.

Arriving home, the boys want to play outside. Andrea opens the garage door so that Carson can get his ramps for his BMX bike. Cooper puts his bike away and gets his basketball. Andrea goes inside the house and gets fresh cold-water bottles for everyone, her book and comes out the front door to sit down on the front steps.

"Boys here's some cold water," she tells them.

"OK" they both reply, and they continue to play.

Andrea smiles watching the boys playing outside in the bright sunshine. She looks around the neighborhood from the front step and sees a few kids playing and she can hear them laughing. A flock of ten Canadian geese in a "v" formation fly overhead honking as they fly by.

Looking down at her watch she sees that it is getting close to lunch. She thinks to herself, *I don't feel like fixing anything for lunch.* So, she asks the Carson and Cooper, "would you guys like to go out to eat lunch?"

"YEAH!" they respond.

"Well, let's put everything away, get cleaned up and head out to the 5-1 Diner," she says to them. The boys put away their stuff and go in through the garage. Andrea meets them inside. They all go upstairs to get ready to go eat.

"I'm ready!" yells Carson as he bounds down the stairs to go get his shoes on.

Cooper is close behind him, "me too!"

Andrea walks down the stairs, gets her shoes on and they all go out and get into her truck.

They head to the 5-1 Diner for lunch, it's a short distance to the next town where it is located. Andrea finds a parking spot in the back-parking lot, as the parking along the building is too short for her truck.

They walk through the park area that is by the diner. The park has a white gazebo on the side by the back-parking lot. It also has a memorial to veterans in the corner by the parking lots. Carson and Cooper run along the sidewalk inside the park and stop as they get to the sidewalk next to the road. Andrea catches up to the boys and they all continue over to the diner.

They enter the diner on the side and get in line for a table. Nicole, the owner, greets them and takes them to a table outside on the patio that faces the busy main street of town. Jenn comes over, gives them menus and says, "What would you like to drink?"

"Root beer" both boys order because it's served in its bottle.

Andrea orders, "I'll have water with lemon."

"I'll be right back with those and take your order," replies Jenn.

A few minutes later Jenn returns with their drinks, "are you ready to order?"

"I want the fish sandwich and fries," Cooper replies.

Carson orders, "I want chewy bacon and hash browns."

Andrea puts the menu down, "I'll have the chicken Caesar wrap."

Jenn takes the menus and says, "I'll get your orders right in."

She goes and puts in their order and comes back out in a few minutes to talk with them. They are regulars.

"So, how are you guys doing?" Jenn asks.

"Great, I started a 5K walking training program. We are at the three-week mark now," Andrea replies.

"Is that the one over in Oakland?"

"Yes, it is. I am enjoying walking with a great group of ladies. Plus, we have homework and I do some of it with the boys. Today we went and did a track workout. Well, I walked, and they rode their bikes."

"Did you boys have fun?"

"Yeah!" they both replied.

"Then we decided to come here for lunch. I love coming here to eat and they love the food and sitting out on the patio watching all the vehicles going by."

"There's a 76 Chevy Corvette," Carson interjects as the car goes by.

"Wow, you really know your cars," Jenn replies.

"Yep, over there is a 70 Ford Mustang."

"Well, I am going to check on other tables and your food."

It isn't very long, and their meals arrive to the table. Everyone gets very quiet while they eat lunch. Jenn arrives back at the table and asks, "do you guys need anything else?"

"No, we are all set for today," replies Andrea.

She leaves the check on the table.

Everyone finishes their lunch. Andrea says, "ready to go boys? We can go play in the park downtown."

"Yeah" they both reply.

Carson and Cooper get up and go inside to the register where they can get suckers. Andrea leaves a tip on the table and follows behind them.

"How was everything?" Nicole asks.

"Excellent, as usual," Andrea replies.

"Glad to hear it. How's everything going?"

"Great, I have started a 5K walking training program in Oakland."

"Well that sounds like fun."

"So far it is."

"Here's your change. Have a great day."

"Thanks, you too. See you later."

"See you later."

They walk back to the truck the same way they walked to the diner. It's a lot safer than going through the parking lot.

Everyone piles into the truck and go to the park in downtown Lake Orion.

The boys see the park, and get big smiles on their faces. Andrea asks them, "are you excited to get out and play with the other kids?"

"Yeah!" they both replied.

They get out of the truck and Carson runs for the swings. "Watch how high I can go this time!" he says.

Cooper runs over to his favorite slide that is built into the side of the hill. Andrea enjoys sitting on the one of the hill seats watching the boys and taking lots of pictures of them.

Andrea says to the boys, "Carson and Cooper, time to go home." They all walk over to the truck and head for home.

Chapter 9: Week 4

It's a cold and drizzly day. Andrea thinks to herself, *I do not want to go to training tonight, however, I am the one bringing the after-walk treats. I have to go.* Andrea gets her Capri black running leggings on and a long sleeve tech shirt. It's cooler tonight then it has been for the other nights plus it's raining, she doesn't want to get chilled.

The doorbell rings and it is Michael. He has come over to watch the boys while Andrea is at training. He is very supportive of her new lifestyle and loves spending more time with the boys.

Carson and Cooper come running to the door. "Dad!" they holler. Carson opens the door for his dad. Both of them give him a big hug as he tries coming inside. He is able to carry them inside as he goes sideways through the front door.

Andrea comes downstairs and gets her shoes on. She gives both the boys a hug and kiss and tells Michael, "there's lasagna in the oven that is only being kept warm, so you guys can eat anytime. Thanks for coming over to watch the boys."

Andrea picks up her cooler of goodies, which are small juice boxes, boxes of raisins and fruit snacks, and leaves in her truck.

As she drives towards Oakland High School North along the road to her right is a deer that is standing there eating the grass, not paying attention to any of the traffic going by. Andrea continues to the school and parks her truck next to Angela's car.

Andrea is the first one there besides Angela.

"Hey, how's it going?" Angela says as Andrea walks up to her.

"Everything's going great, you?" Andrea replies.

"Wonderful. I am excited for tonight's walk. Although, I am excited about every night's walk."

Gradually everyone arrives and comes over to Angela's car. "Hi everyone. Tonight's walk will be a 30-minute walk. We will go on the path along Tienken over to Squirrel and a little bit up Squirrel and then back. You gals have been doing a great job of getting over for other groups and encouraging them. Plus, I hope you all have been keeping up on your homework. It is so important for your progress. Let's get moving!" Angela encourages everyone.

They head out on the path along the school. The route is along a two-lane road, so there is some traffic but not like it was when they were training along University. Angela hollers out "arms up" and "arms down" according to her fitness watch prompts.

They have been out for a few minutes or so and Angela says, "let's do something different with our arms up, this time we will go single file and the person at the back will walk as fast as they can to the front of the line, when they get to the front of the line they will say "Next" and then the next person at the back will go to the front of the line and follow suit until everyone has been able to go to the front of the group from the back of the group. I will start us off. Single file and arms up!"

Angela puts her arms up at the 90-degree angle and walks quickly to the front of the group and says "Next!" which is Andrea who walks quickly to the front of the group and says "Next" and it continues with Vickie, Kim, Karin, Denese, Doree and finally Sharon gets to the front of the group but says "Last one!" to indicate that she is the last of the group.

"How did you all like that game?" asks Angela.

"Loved it!" replied Andrea, Karin and Vickie

"It was fun!" replied Denese, Doree, Kim and Sharon.

"Glad to hear it. We will do this to shake things up a bit when there's room on the path or trail we are on. Ok, time to get back on track with arms down." Angela tells the group.

Next, they come alongside the gated community, pass by the gated entrance where there is a white guard house with white gate arms that are down blocking traffic. Inside the guard house is a little old man reading a paper patiently waiting for people to come up to the gate.

After the gated community the group comes to the intersection of Tienken and Squirrel. The group goes to the right on Squirrel, so they don't have to worry about crossing the road. They go as far as the condo complex road and turn around.

Angela says, "Ok, let's turn around and this we will have the ones at the back of the group lead the group back to Tienken."

When they get to Tienken the group turns left and heads toward the school. Angela is at the front of the group and sees another group headed their way. "Runners Up! Single file!" she instructs the group. They meet up with the runners and give them a high five and encouraging words of "great job!" "keep it up" "lookin' good!"

A few more minutes and they are at Angela's car and Andrea gets her cooler out of her truck and places it in the back of Angela's car. "I must say you ladies are doing a great job of walking and must all be doing your homework; our pace is nice and we are staying close together. Tonight's goodies are from Andrea and she brought small juice boxes, boxes of raisins and fruit snacks. I want to remind everyone that the stretching exercises can actually be done every day if you like. This will really help with your muscles. Now next week we are going to be meeting back down at the library and parking in the same area we did last week. I will have a different route for us to take. Next week's goodies will be brought by Karin. Does anyone have any questions or comments?" Angela asks.

Everyone looks at each other and shakes their head no. "Ok, I will see everyone next week then." Says Angela.

"See you next week," everyone replies.

Andrea picks up her cooler, puts it in her truck. She heads for home to see her boys. Andrea thinks to herself I am really glad that the training program locations are so close to home.

She gets home, pulls into the garage and goes inside. As she opens the door Andrea hollers, "boys, I am home!"

The boys come running to the door to give her a big hug and kiss.

Michael gets up off the couch and gets his shoes on. He says to the boys, "It's been a fun evening and I'll see you tomorrow. Get some sleep." The boys both give him a hug good bye. Michael leaves out the front door.

Andrea takes her shoes off and says to the boys, "time for bed boys, go upstairs and get ready."

Cooper and Carson run upstairs and get ready for bed. Andrea takes her cooler to the kitchen, places it on the table, empties it out and goes upstairs.

The boys are all ready and get into their own beds. She goes in and gives them each a hug and kiss good night. She heads to her room and gets her pajamas on, lays down and reads for a while before going to sleep.

Chapter 10: Weather Doesn't Cooperate

It's another beautiful day outside, the sky is just starting to get a few clouds in it. Andrea is sitting at the dining room table on her laptop while Cooper and Carson are in the living room watching Scooby Doo. She says to the boys, "You guys want to go to a park and ride your bikes?"

"Yeah!" they reply, Carson turns off the tv and they get their shoes on.

Andrea puts her shoes on and they go in the garage, put their bikes in the back of the truck under the tonneau cover and get in her truck.

They get about half way to the park; the clouds open and the rains starts coming down in buckets. She turns her windshield wipers on high. Previously Andrea would have just turned the truck around and gone home. However, this time she says to the boys, "bummer it's raining, guess we will go to the mall instead of the park.

Carson responds, "awe man!"

Andrea turns at the next intersection to go in the direction of the mall instead of the park. Cooper had fallen asleep in the truck and wakes up, looking out the window and sees the mall. "What are we doing here?" asks Cooper.

"With it raining we have to walk in the mall," replies Andrea. She finds a parking space, parks the truck and says to the boys, "All right boys, let's get out on one side of the truck, take my hands and let's run inside."

They get out of their seats, Andrea opens the door and they jump out, take her hands and run inside with the rain pouring down and splashing in the puddles along the way.

They make it under the overhang and go in through the glass and wood doors that have antler door handles. The boys let go of her hands and run over to the huge towering stone fireplace with a roaring fire. Andrea is close behind them, reaches out and takes both of their hands.

"Come on boys, let's get going. If you boys are good while walking in the mall we will come back and go on the pontoon boats and four-wheelers," she says to them.

The boys cooperate and walk with her through the turnstile entrance, saying hello to the elderly gentleman greeter. Walking straight ahead they go to the 23,000-gallon fish tank and make faces at the fish swimming around the tank.

"Let's get moving boys," she says to them and tugs on their hands. Going around the corner they come across the race car display and Cooper must stop and look at everything. Andrea lightly tugs on Cooper's hand and they continue to the large wood and glass doors that go out into the mall.

Going to the right and staying to the right the boys continue to hold Andrea's hands. Cooper must slow down in front of all the shoe stores.

They stop at the pretzel store and she tells them, "we can stop another time."

Both boys make disappointed faces but continue walking. They walk down all the entrance hallways.

Passing by the ice cream stand they all take a deep sniff of the freshly baked waffle cones.

Andrea and the boys continue to the right.

"This store has basketball shoes and jerseys," comments Cooper.

"And this one too," he continues as they go by another store.

The one corridor has only a couple of people in it and the boys start skipping. As they turn the corner out of the corridor they switch back to walking and Carson pulls Andrea and Cooper along towards the white Dodge Ram 1500 that is sitting in the middle of the hallway.

Cooper then pulls them towards the arcade place with all the bright flashing lights and video game sounds. "Ok guys let's slow down a bit. We have to watch where we are going. Also, we are not going into the arcade today."

A short distance from the arcade is Building Blocks Discovery Center and the boys love looking at all the different Lego building sets. It's a slow walk through the store area.

"Can we go inside?" the boys ask.

"Not today, but we will be back," replies Andrea. She tugs on their hands and they follow her out of the store and continuing to the right.

Rounding the bend there is a strong smell of popcorn in the air as they walk closer to the movie theater. The sign with 14 different movies comes into view. They walk close to the theater, see all the boxes of candy and take in the freshly popped popcorn smell. No Scooby Doo movies at this time, just new movies. The boys frown in disappointment.

Continuing along the right side of the mall they come to the alligator in the front of Gator Land Cafe. Cooper walks close by the mouth and the alligator opens his mouth and roars, Cooper jumps back a few inches and Carson laughs. "Come on boys, let's continue on," Andrea says to them.

Following along to the right they come to the Aquarium. The boys are excited to see the small aquarium in the front area.

Carson says, "We want to go in."

"Boys, we will come back here another day. Today we are just walking inside the mall," replies Andrea. After a few moments of looking at the fish in the aquarium Andrea tugs on the boys' hands and they go with her down the hallway of the mall looking in the windows of the stores.

The carousel is on their left as they reach the food court area and they can hear the Calliope music. Andrea takes the boys over to the carousel, buys them tickets and they get in line. The carousel is going around counter clockwise and slowly comes to a stop. The children and adults get off the carousel and the attendant opens the gate for everyone to enter.

Carson goes to the brown horse while Cooper goes to a white horse. Andrea sits in the chariot that is being pulled by a dolphin. The other children and adults are going to their choices of where to sit. The attendant closes the gate, walks around the carousel taking the tickets from all the passengers and starts the carousel going. It goes around for two minutes with the horses going up and down, the teacup spinning around in circles and the dolphins going back and forth. The carousel slowly comes to a stop, the attendant opens the gate, and everyone gets off.

Cooper says, "that was fun!"

"Yeah!" Carson agrees.

"Alright, let's continue on," replies Andrea.

As they walk back into the hallway the smell of fresh popped popcorn is filling the air. "Boys, how would you like some popcorn?" Andrea asks them.

"Yeah!" they both reply.

"Ok, we will get some and take it home with us to watch Scooby Doo. Remember on our way out we are going to get on the boats and four-wheelers," Andrea informs them.

Carson picks out a bag of butter flavored popcorn. Cooper chooses the caramel corn and Andrea picks out the kettle corn.

Across from the popcorn stand is the store where they came in. Going back into the store they go through the turnstile. They walk up on the wood plank bridge that crosses over the duck pond where a waterwheel is turning and water cascades down into the pond containing bright orange Koi fish.

Carson leads the way to the left where they walk through the fishing department and get to the pontoon boats that are on display. He walks up the stairs to get onto the pontoon. Carson sits down in the captain's chair, Cooper sits at the back on the lounger and Andrea takes pictures of the boys. There are three different styles of pontoon boats and the boys must go on all three of them.

Across from the pontoons are the four-wheelers, Carson jumps down from the pontoon boat and gets up on a bright red four-wheeler. Cooper runs over and gets into a bright lime green four-seater ATV. "I want this one!" he says.

"Yeah, I'll get right on that Cooper!" Andrea says to him as she reads the price tag and sees it's over $20,000. "You better start saving your pennies," she jokingly tells him.

Carson comes over and gets in the passenger seat. "I like it too!" he says.

"You guys are killing me," she laughs. "Ok boys, time to head home." They climb out of the four-seater ATV and take her hands.

They get to the doors to go outside; the sun is shining, and the clouds have dispersed. "Alright! This is awesome. When we get home you guys can play outside." Andrea tells the boys.

"Yeah!" they reply and walk, holding Andrea's hands, to the truck.

Arriving home Andrea pulls the truck in the garage and everyone gets out of the truck. Carson grabs his bike and Cooper gets his basketball. The boys are playing, smiling and laughing in the warmth and sunshine. Andrea takes the bags of popcorn inside, sets them on the kitchen table, grabs her tablet and sits down on the front porch to watch the boys and read her eBook.

"Mom is it time for dinner? I am hungry!" Cooper asks.

Looking down at her watch, "yes, it is. What would you like?"

"I want macaroni and cheese!" interjects Carson.

"Yeah, I want that too!" says Cooper.

"Ok, get everything put away and we'll have macaroni and cheese," Andrea tells them.

Getting up she picks up her tablet and goes inside. The boys put their bike and basketball away and go in through the garage.

In the kitchen, Andrea gets out two boxes of macaroni and cheese, two half sticks of butter and coconut milk. She gets the water boiling for the macaroni and Carson pops into the kitchen, "how can I help?"

"After the macaroni cooks I'll need help putting the ingredients in and stirring," she tells him. Then she empties the boxes of macaroni into the boiling water.

"I want to help too!" says Cooper as he slides into the kitchen.

"You can help too."

The macaroni is done, Andrea drains the water off of the macaroni and dumps the macaroni into a large mixing bowl. She thinks to herself *this will give enough room for the boys to mix in the ingredients.*

"Ok boys, who wants to mix and who wants to put the ingredients in?" she asks them.

"I want to mix," Carson says quickly before Cooper can reply.

"So, here's the bowl of macaroni and the big wooden spoon," she says as she places them in front of Carson at the table.

"Cooper, I will hand you the ingredients and you will put them in the bowl while Carson stirs."

She hands Cooper the first stick of butter, "you have to unwrap it and put it in the bowl."

Cooper unwraps the stick of butter and drops it in the bowl. Carson stirs the macaroni and stick of butter. The heat of the macaroni melts the butter.

"Here's the next stick," Andrea hands Cooper the butter. He unwraps it and drops it into the bowl.

"Next we have the coconut milk," she says as she pours the coconut milk into a measuring cup and hands it to Cooper.

Cooper pours the milk over the macaroni and butter.

"The last thing we have is the powdered cheese," she tears open the packet and hands it to Cooper.

Cooper dumps the powder out and into the bowl. Carson is continuing to mix everything together.

Taking the bowl and spoon from Carson she says, "Ok, you guys get the bowls and spoons and set them on the table."

As they are setting the bowls and spoons on the table Andrea gives the macaroni and cheese a few more stirs to make sure it's all mixed together thoroughly. She takes the bowl of macaroni and cheese to the table and spoons it into the bowls.

They all sit down to the table and eat dinner. The boys are quiet because they are eating.

"After dinner we can watch a movie and eat popcorn. How does that sound?" she asks them.

"Yeah!" says Cooper.

"Sounds good," says Carson.

Their bowls are empty, and the boys get up from the table and put their bowls and spoons in the dishwasher. Andrea cleans up the rest of the kitchen.

Walking into the living room with the bags of popcorn she sees the boys have already turned on the tv and put in a movie. It's a car movie. They all snuggle on the couch, eating their popcorn and watch the movie.

Chapter 11: Week 5

The training program is at the half way point as they head into week 5. Andrea is sitting in the living room looking at her schedule to see that they have a 30 minute walk this evening. The boys are sitting on the floor watching their favorite tv show, Scooby Doo. She looks down at her fitness watch, sees that it's time to go and says to the boys, "time to go to your dad's, go get your shoes on."

Cooper says, "I want to go walk with you mom."

Andrea says "Sorry Cooper, but you can't go with me tonight. We'll go for a walk tomorrow. Go get your shoes on."

"Ok," he replies.

They all get in her truck and head over to Michael's. Carson points out the window, "look at the ducks!" as they drive by the pond with the ducks.

Andrea pulls up in Michael's driveway and he is sitting out on his front porch. Michael waves hello as they pull up. Cooper and Carson get out of the truck and go up on the front porch. Andrea gets out of the truck, gives the boys each a hug and kiss, then gets back into her truck. They boys and Michael wave good-bye as she backs out of the driveway and then she drives to the library to meet her walking group.

Upon arrival Andrea sees Angela's car and pulls into the parking spot next to her. Vickie is also there. Andrea, Angela and Vickie hang out by Angela's car.

"Hi!" Angela says as Andrea walks up.

"Hi!" Andrea says.

"Hello!" replies Vickie.

"How's the walking going?" Angela asks.

"I am enjoying it. I have taken the boys with me. In fact, the boys ride their bikes as I walk," says Angela with a smile.

The rest of the group joins them in a few minutes.

Angela informs her group of ladies, "We are going to go out and go to the right. We will go on the trail behind the library and follow it along to tie into the Clinton River trail. Then we will turn around and head back here to have treats that Karin brought. Ready?"

"Ready!" replies everyone.

"Arms up and let's go!" Angela yells.

They start off walking on the trail that goes along the creek behind the library. They stay single file as the trail is busy with a lot of people out for a walk, run or bike ride.

Andrea is at the front of the group and they come to their first road crossing. This one is very well marked and even has a sign that says that pedestrians have the right of way. The road is a small two-lane road and this crossing is at the bottom of a small curvy hill. It is not a super busy road, as it is off the main road by a block or so. The ladies can cross the road with no traffic.

The trail goes between an independent living community and the creek. The maple trees create a canopy over the trail; they walk by the creek and hear the water running through the rocks. They get to a bridge and cross over the creek. The trail continues alongside the creek and comes out at a road where the ladies must stop and wait for the traffic to stop.

Once they cross the small busy road they are now on a sidewalk across from some businesses. They pick up the Clinton River Trail at the end of the sidewalk.

Angela tells the group, "we are going to the right and we'll turn around when we get to the large Main Street bridge that will be overhead. How is everyone doing?"

"Great" they all reply.

"We are going to follow the trail to the left and go along by the river." Angela tells her group.

"This is a fairly new section of the trail, previously it went straight." Even though they are in the busy downtown area they can hear the river flowing over the rocks and the ducks quacking.

During their walk the ladies are talking the whole way amongst themselves. They are getting to know each other on a personal level.

"I have 5-year-old twin boys, Carson and Cooper. Carson likes to ride his BMX bike and Cooper likes to play basketball. What about you?" Andrea asks Karin.

Karin replies, "My kids are grown. I have a boy and a girl and 7 grandkids. My husband passed away 5 years ago, and I took up walking with the training group to meet people."

"I am a computer programmer. I sit at a desk all day staring at a computer screen. It's great to get out and walk and talk with people," Kim says to Vickie.

"Crazy thing is I am on my feet all day with being a nurse, but it's so much more fun to be walking with people outside," Vickie replies to Kim.

"What have you been up to at work?" Sharon asks Doree.

"Same ol', same ol'. Nothing much exciting, which I guess is something good these days," Doree replies.

"Denese, how are your feet this year?" Angela asks.

"They are doing really well. I went to Bauman's Running and Walking store. They fitted me with a great pair of shoes. They are so comfy. I love them," replies Denese.

Staying to the right on the trail the group gets to the overhead Main Street bridge and then loop down to the creek. There is a boat ramp where one can launch a canoe or kayak. The ladies are now on their return trip of their walk. This time when they cross the road back along the creek they go straight instead of crossing the bridge. The trail goes up along a local luxury hotel and they take the sidewalk to the crosswalk. The ducks are splashing and quacking in the creek.

The group makes their way around the back of the library and back to Angela's car where Karin gets the goodies out of her car and brings them over to Angela's. "We did a great pace tonight ladies. We are already half way through the program. We only have 4 more weeks of training and then it's race time. You should have received an email detailing how you register on-line. If you have any questions, please let me know and I can help you. Now is the time to get a new pair of shoes if you didn't get them before the training program. Also, start figuring out what you are going to wear the morning of the race. Remember that the race is on July 4th, so it will be a very warm if not just down right hot the morning of the race. It's also a great time to try out what you'll be having for breakfast before the race. Do this on Saturday mornings for your walk homework. Let's enjoy the wonderful grapes and bottles of water that Karin brought us tonight." Angela says to the group.

"What do you recommend for breakfast before a race?" asks Denese.

"There are a few options that people do. One is a bowl of oatmeal with their favorite toppings like raisins and/or nuts. Others eat protein bars and bananas. Another option is a protein smoothie with fruit in it," replies Angela.

"Any other questions?" Angela asks.

"No" the ladies respond.

"Next week we will meet over at Castlebury. It is on Joslyn Rd just north of Waldon. We will meet in the parking lot by the first entrance on the south end. We will finish up at Yates at Canterbury where we will have cider and donuts or cider slushes for a special treat. See you ladies next week!" Angela informs the group.

Andrea gets into her truck and drives over to Michael's to get her boys. She is thankful for the short drive over to her ex's after training. She pulls into his driveway, gets out of her truck and goes up to the door. Andrea rings the doorbell and the boys come running to the door to greet her.

"Cooper! Carson! Ready?" she says. The boys come outside, and Michael is following behind them with their bags.

"Here you go boys. I'll see you later." Carson and Cooper give Michael a hug and kiss goodbye.

Carson, Cooper and Andrea get into her truck and drive the short distance home. Everyone piles out of the truck, goes inside the townhouse and gets ready for bed.

Chapter 12: Walk in the Park

Andrea pulls into a parking space. The boys are looking out their windows, "where are we?" they ask.

"We are in a park that I used to go to when I was growing up," she replies. They get out of the truck and Andrea takes the boys' bikes out of the back of the truck.

Carson and Cooper ride their bikes over to the play structure. Leaning their bikes against the fence they run to the ladders and climb up, run across to the winding tube slide and go down the slides feet first. The boys go up and down and all around the play structure, climbing, running and sliding for 30 minutes.

"All right boys let's check out the rest of the park," Andrea says to the boys.

The boys get on their bikes and follow behind Andrea as they leave the play structure area and go to the concrete path that follows the creek. The path leads under the road where the water in the creek runs over and around a large number of rocks of various sizes. As traffic drives above them the noise echoes around them. On their right as they come out from the overpass there is a skatepark.

"Can I go ride over there mom?" asks Carson.

Andrea replies, "Sorry bud, the sign says no bikes. Let's keep moving."

Cooper gets off his bike and walks it near the creek where he points out the fish that are swimming. Carson decides to get off his bike too.

Andrea says to them, "come on boys, let's pick up the pace a little bit." They both get back on their bikes and start peddling to get ahead of Andrea.

They come to a steel tunnel under the next road. The boys love it as they are able to make all kinds of loud noises. Making their way through the tunnel they come out the other side where the sun is shining above them and the grass is a vivid green. In the distance they hear a clickety clack sound, it keeps getting louder and then a train horn is blowing.

"Yeah! A train!" both boys exclaim.

"Let's stay here and wait for the train to go by," says Andrea. As they sit on their bikes the train comes into view and quickly moves along the tracks.

Carson counts out loud, "one, two, three, four, five, six..." and continues to count all the cars. He gets to the end, "fifty-two, fifty-two cars!"

Andrea says to the boys, "Ok, we will go through this next tunnel and turn around and go back the other way."

Carson takes off on his bike through the tunnel followed closely behind by Cooper. They wait on the other side of the tunnel for Andrea to catch up. When she catches up, they turn around, head back through the tunnel and pedal quickly to the next tunnel where they stop before going through and, again, wait for Andrea to catch up.

Andrea finally rejoins the boys and they all continue through the steel tunnel.

"AAAHHHHH!" yells Carson

"YEAH!" yells Cooper

"Woohoo!" yells Carson

"AAAAHHHHHH!" yells Cooper

They smile listening to the echo.

Near the skate park is a train made out of steel tubes that the boys can climb and hang, Cooper races to the train on his bike, lays his bike down and climbs onto the train. Carson follows him and does the same thing.

Andrea thinks to herself *I am glad to see them climbing on the train. It gives me time to catch up to my boys.*

She brings out her camera and takes a bunch of pictures of the boys playing on the train. They make all kinds of silly and happy faces for her.

"Hey boys, let's go back to the truck and we can make a special stop on the way home," Andrea says.

"Alright!" both boys jump down off the train, get on their bikes and pedal full speed to the bridge where they both come to abrupt stops because there are people under the bridge and they need to wait for Andrea to catch up.

She catches up to the boys and says, "get off your bikes and walk them past the people that are under the bridge. On the other side of the bridge you can get back on your bikes and ride behind me on the sidewalk."

The park is now filled with kids swinging, riding bikes, and running around while their parents are in the pavilions setting up for dinner and talking. Andrea then sees a big Coach bus and a black Chevrolet truck with a black enclosed trailer. Sitting next to the trailer is a black Corvette. The banner on the chain link fence reads "Big & Rich."

Andrea asks the boys, "hey, you guys want to stay and listen to some great music?"

"Yeah!" they reply.

"Ok, let's go back to the truck to get a blanket," she tells them.

The boys race to the truck and Carson gets there first. "I win!" he yells.

Cooper is close behind him. Andrea joins them at the truck, she puts the tailgate down and loads the bikes into the back of the truck. Cooper gets the blanket out of the backseat and Carson gets the cooler and wheels it across the parking lot.

On the grass close by the creek Cooper lays down the blanket. Carson stops with the cooler on the edge of the blanket and they all get their spot on the blanket. In the cooler are cans of Phyzix Zero, a natural energy drink that they all love. Other goodies include boxes of Mike and Ike's including their favorite flavors: Berry Blast, Tropical Typhoon and Hot Tamales; barbecue chips, regular chips, carrot sticks and a choice of peanut butter sandwiches made with grape jelly or apple cinnamon jelly.

They are enjoying their picnic dinner on the blanket next to the creek where the ducks are swimming and quaking. As the band starts playing they sing along and watch the sunset over the trees.

The sun has set, the band is still playing, and the boys are starting to get tired. Carson is rubbing his eyes and Cooper is laying down on the blanket.

"Come on boys, let's get going," Andrea tells the boys.

They put all the stuff in the cooler and Cooper gets up and wraps the blanket around himself. Andrea holds each of their hands and Carson pulls the cooler back to the truck.

She gets the boys in their seats, gets in the truck herself and slowly drives out of the park, watching for people crossing the road and opening vehicle doors along the road.

"How would you boys like to stop for a treat?" Andrea asks.

"Yeah!" they both reply.

"Ok, we are going to stop at the Caboose for ice cream!"

"I want superman!" replies Carson.

"I want blue moon!" replies Cooper.

"Alright, sounds good."

They drive to the Caboose. She parks right in front, they get out and go up to the window.

"How can I help you?" Carrie asks.

"I want superman!" Carson tells her.

"Kids superman for him and kids blue moon for this one," she says pointing to Cooper.

"And I will have a kid's blueberry soft serve cone for myself."

Andrea pays for the cones. The kids get their cones first and then she has her cone. They all sit at the red rectangular picnic table.

"Ok boys, time to go," she tells them as they finish their cones. The boys get into their seats in the truck and Andrea gets into her seat. Driving home the boys fall asleep.

Chapter 13: Week 6

It's Thursday afternoon and Andrea receives a phone call from Michael, "Sorry I am going to be late getting the boys tonight. Can I meet you at your group meeting location?"

"Yes, we are meeting at Castlebury on Joslyn Rd north of Waldon Rd. We start walking at 6:30 pm. So, you'll need to be there by 6:30 pm." Andrea replies.

"Ok, I'll be there." Michael promises.

Looking at the clock, Andrea says to the boys, "Carson, Cooper, it's time to go. Your dad is going to meet us there. Get your stuff and get in the truck."

The boys get up, turn off the tv, put their shoes on and head out to the truck. Andrea follows right behind them.

This time the ride is even shorter as they live less than a mile from Castlebury. The boys smile as they are going here they say, "I hope dad will let us stay and eat dinner at the C-Pub. We love the pizza there."

Upon arrival at Castlebury Andrea she sees that only Angela is there so far. Andrea pulls up next to Angela. She gets out of her truck and says to Angela, "my ex is coming to get the boys and has promised to be here before 6:30."

Angela tells her, "don't worry we'll wait for him."

The boys get out of the truck and say, "hi!" and stay near Andrea.

Sharon, Karin, Kim and Vickie come over and Andrea says, "ladies, these are my boys, Carson and Cooper. Boys say hi."

"Hi!" they both reply.

Just then Michael pulls up next to Andrea's truck. As soon as Michael opens his door Carson goes running over, followed closely by Cooper. He hugs the boys and asks them, "do you guys want to eat at the C-Pub?"

"YEAH!!!" they responded. Carson takes Michael's hand and Cooper takes his other hand.

Michael and the boys walk over to the C-Pub and sit on the outdoor patio. They walk up to the hostess station, "Welcome. Would you like to sit inside or outside on the patio?"

"We'd like to sit at a table by the edge of the patio, so they can see their mom go by on her walk."

"Follow me," the hostess says.

The sit down and the waitress comes up to the table.

"What would you like to drink?" ask the waitress.

"We'll have a pitcher of Sierra Mist and we are ready to order our dinner also," Michael says.

"Ok, what would you like?"

"We'll have a pizza with pepperoni, mushrooms, Italian sausage, ham, bacon and ground beef along with a large antipasto salad."

"Thank you, I'll get that ordered and bring your Sierra Mist out first."

"Yeah! Our favorite!" the boys cheer.

The rest of Angela's walking group finally arrives. Angela begins, "Ok ladies, tonight we are doing laps around Castlebury. This is going to be fun. There's a nice incline shortly after we get started, we'll go past the C-Pub where you can smell the food cooking, then we will go along the front of the castle, around the church and back to here. We will probably do three laps. Then we will finish at Yates at Canterbury for our post workout treat. Everyone ready?!"

"Yes!" they reply.

Angela leads the group of ladies onto Joslyn Ct and up the slight incline leading them in front of a cluster of little houses painted in primary colors; each house filled with unique items for sale. Next, they go by the C-Pub and they all wave to Carson and Cooper who are standing just inside the patio area.

"Hi mom!" they both yell.

"Hi!" the group says back to them.

They go right around the end of the C-Pub where it is a short distance to go around to the front of the castle. It's an old-world style castle with the large pillars. The parking lot is lined with pine trees along the roadside. There are lots of twinkling white lights in the trees.

There is lots of room for them to walk and they spread out chatting and allowing more of them in the conversation.

They get to the entrance of the church parking lot and Angela says, "let's pick it up and see how fast we can go to the entrance by our vehicles."

Everyone picks up the pace. Andrea and Vickie take the lead as they go around the corner of the church. They maintain the lead to the parking lot entrance with Kim and Denese hot on their tails. They take a short break until the rest of the group joins them at the entrance.

"First lap down ladies. Great job!" remarks Angela. "Let's see how long it takes us for this next lap."

They head out on their second lap, taking note of the carousel house and observing that it's open and going around. All the ladies wave and say, "Hi Carson and Cooper!"

Cooper and Carson wave from their table on the patio of the C-Pub.

This time along the front of the castle they do their "leapfrog" of having the last person walk quickly to the front of the single file line. Sharon is at the back of the line and starts everyone off. They go through the line twice along the front of the castle and church.

Making their way to the end of their second lap they all shout, "Two laps down!"

Then continuing to start their third lap. This time they mix it up with taking the path behind Yates at Canterbury to the front of the village and head past the front of the castle and then coming around the end of the C-Pub they wave to Carson and Cooper on the patio.

"Hi Mom!" they yell.

"Hi!" the ladies all yell back.

The boys finish up their pizza and Sierra Mist. The waitress brings the bill and Michael pays with cash. They get up and head towards Yates at Canterbury.

The ladies head back towards Yates at Canterbury following the path to the front going along the front of the church and returning back to their vehicles.

Once back at their vehicles they all cheer, "DONE!!!" and then walk up to Yates at Canterbury for their post workout treat of cider and donuts.

They all go inside.

"Can I help you?" says Megan, the lady working behind the counter.

"I'll have a cider slush," says Sharon.

"Can I help you?" Mark asks from behind the counter.

"I'll also have a cider slush," says Karin.

"How many of you are having cider slushes?" asks Paula, who is also behind the counter.

The rest of the ladies raise their hands.

"Ok, everyone can line up at the register and I'll get the slushes."

Megan takes Sharon's cider slush to the register and Sharon pays her.

As they get their slushes and pay, they go and sit down in the table area.

Then Michael comes in with Carson and Cooper. The boys run up to Andrea and give her a big hug. They sit down at the next table while Michael goes up to the counter.

"Can I help you?" asks Mark.

"Yes, I'll have a cider slush and two small blue moon ice cream cones," Michael replies.

He gets his order and sits down with the boys.

While the walkers are seated together and enjoying their goodies Angela says, "next week we will have a 60-minute walk in Kent Lake Park. We will park at the first parking lot at the East Boat Launch. This will get us some nice rolling hills. Bring your sunscreen. I will see you all next week."

"See you next week," they all reply.

After a few minutes the ladies leave.

Andrea says to the boys, "let's head home."

Cooper is done with his ice cream and Carson is almost done with his. Carson finishes his ice cream and they all get up and walk back to the trucks.

Michael gives the boys hugs and kisses. "See you later guys." He gets in his truck and goes home.

Andrea gets the boys into their seats in her truck and they head home.

Chapter 14: Trip to Little Bavaria

The view outside the truck's passenger window as they approach the town is a landscape of various Christmas decorations: nativity scene, candy canes, reindeer, ornaments, packages, lighted arches, Santa and more. Andrea rolls down the window and they hear Christmas carols. It is the world's largest Christmas store.

"Can we go there mom?" the boys ask.

"Not today, we are going to walk around downtown. We'll go there another day," replies Andrea.

Around the bend and a short distance down the road out through the driver's side window Carson spots a bunch of trucks that are being displayed for the local dealership. "There's a Dodge Ram, a Jeep Wrangler, a Dodge Charger, a Fiat 124 Spider and a Jeep Compass," Carson informs them.

On the right and down the road is a Bavarian style shopping area called River Shops. Andrea turns into the parking lot on the south end of the shops and finds a parking spot. The boys are so excited, they are quickly out of their seats and jump down out of the truck. Andrea puts a bracelet on each boy that has a spiral cable attached which in turn Andrea attaches to her wrists. Carson's is blue, and Cooper's is orange.

Before crossing the roadway in the parking lot, they look both ways, no cars coming, and they walk over to the entrance of the River Shops. It is a three-story tower with arches and walkways on four sides. On the other side of the entrance they follow the path to the right. There are all kinds of stores: a mirror maze, a bakery, a store that has items made in Michigan, an ice cream shop and many more.

At the north end of the shops there's a bridge that crosses the river. They start across the bridge and stop at the first balcony to check out the waterfall that goes down the hill from the shops to the river with water cascading down over rocks. Not too far from the waterfall is a riverboat that people are boarding, and they listen to the Dixieland music that is playing on the riverboat.

Cooper is checking out the flags that are displayed on the bridge, "United States, Canada, France, Germany, Italy and I don't know the rest."

Andrea says to the boys, "come on let's keep going. We'll walk up one side, come back the other side and finish up with dinner at the Bavarian Inn Restaurant."

They get off the bridge and there's a Bavarian style gift shop, they slow down to look in the windows and see all the town themed tourist gifts. At the traffic light located at the north end of the gift shop they stop for the red light and watch as the black horse and white carriage comes thru the wooden covered bridge onto the main road listening to the horses' hooves click on the road. The light changes and both boys grab Andrea's hands and cross the street. The Bavarian Inn Restaurant that they will be eating at is on their right. As they walk in front of the restaurant the Glockenspiel plays, and the figures go around.

Continuing on the sidewalk, the boys hold Andrea's hands and stop at the driveways to parking lots to stop and watch for traffic. They walk up to the Maypole water fountain and Carson and Cooper laugh as they splash their hands in the water.

The next store that they stop in front of is the Taffy Shop. They watch the taffy being kissed and pulled by machine in the window. The door opens, and they can smell the fudge that is being poured onto a marble slab.

"Can we get some fudge?" Carson asks.

"Yes, we will get three flavors," Andrea replies, and they go into the Taffy Shop.

The lady behind the counter asks, "which flavors would you like?"

"We'd like the peanut butter fudge, chocolate raspberry fudge and chocolate fudge."

She says, "You get a fourth flavor for free."

"We would like vanilla fudge."

They leave the Taffy Shop and walk to the Cheese Shop next door. There are samples of salsas, jellies, and cheese all around the shop that they happily sample and enjoy. Outside the Cheese Shop is a large statue of a wedge of cheese with a mouse head sticking out of it.

Andrea takes off their bracelets and says, "Stand next to the statue so I can take your picture." Carson and Cooper make all kinds of funny faces and one smile for their pictures.

They put their bracelets back on and continue on up the hill where the sidewalk leads to the front of the brewery. Andrea and the boys walk to the courtyard of the brewery. Andrea takes the boys' bracelets off and takes a photo in front of a large wagon.

Putting their bracelets back on they walk to corner where the traffic light is.

Andrea holds the boys' hands as they cross the street. At the corner is a veteran's memorial park that they walk through before proceeding down the sidewalk. She continues to hold their hands because there are several driveways to cross.

Carson and Cooper slow down in front of another fudge and taffy store. The door opens and, again, the smell of freshly poured hot fudge comes wafting out. They all take a big sniff. Andrea says to the boys, "let's go."

Walking along the sidewalk past various stores the sidewalks are more crowded than they were when they were on the other side. They pass by various restaurants that have outdoor eating where people are sitting and talking. On the left they are at the brick sidewalk that zig zags across the main road. Carson and Cooper are bouncing up and down on their toes while they wait for the light to change anticipating they get to eat soon.....they have spotted The Bavarian Inn Restaurant.

The light changes, they cross the street, go up the brick stairs and walk into the Bavarian Inn Restaurant. They eait themselves in the casual dining area called the Michigan on Main Bar & Grill. Today is a beautiful sunny day and around 70 degrees so Andrea takes the boys to a table on the patio by the sidewalk so that Carson can watch the vehicles go by.

Kelly, their waitress, asks them, "What would you like to drink?"

The boys respond, "root beer" and Andrea replies, "a lemon lime pop."

Kelly returns with their beverages and asks, "are you ready to order?"

Carson and Cooper both say, "the brat and pretzel."

Andrea says, "I'll have the Main Chicken dark."

"Thank you, I'll get that in right away."

Carson is watching the vehicles go by and says, "look a 69 Camaro and a Mustang. Oh look, there's a Harley. I like the cool color of blue on it."

Cooper is drawing on his placemat a race course and driving his die-cast cars on it. Andrea takes pictures of the boys and some of the vehicles that Carson names off.

The food arrives. The boys both exclaim "WOW!" at seeing the size of the brat.

Andrea helps them with cutting the brat into more manageable sizes. Andrea smiles as she looks at her chicken plate, as it is a leg and thigh, Asian salad and potato cheese puffs.

"Do you want anything else?" asks Kelly.

"No, we are all set. Thanks," replies Andrea.

Kelly sets the bill down on the table, "ok, I'll leave this here, no rush."

Andrea pulls out her credit card and rewards card and hands them with the bill to Kelly.

"I'll be right back."

A few moments later Kelly returns, "just sign one copy and have a great day."

"Have a great day," Andrea replies, signs the credit card receipt and puts her cards away in her purse.

"Ok boys let's get going." They get up and walk outside.

Out in the parking lot is an area that is blocked off for a band and they are playing various Polka songs with an accordion, a couple of clarinets, a couple trumpets, a saxophone, a keyboard and a drum set. They walk into the parking lot where the polka band is playing and do some dancing.

Continuing on they walk over to the wooden covered bridge and in the middle of the bridge they stop and look down at the river and the riverboat as it goes under the bridge and has to collapse its smoke towers to clear the bridge.

"Let's take a selfie," she tells the boys. They get a picture with the river in the background.

Moving along on the bridge they walk towards their truck. The truck is parked on the other side of the River Shops. Andrea takes hold of their hands and locates their truck.

"We have made it back. Time to get up in your seats. You guys look tired."

"I am," says Cooper.

"Not me," Carson insists.

She puts both the boys in their seats, gets in her truck and heads for home. Both boys are sleeping within minutes of pulling out of the parking lot. Andrea has a very quiet ride home.

Chapter 15: Week 7

Andrea is so excited to go walking at Kent Lake Park. She gives the boys a hug and kiss goodbye and then drives from their dad's home to Kent Lake Park. This is a slightly longer drive, but it will be a great workout with the changes in terrain.

A nice drive later Andrea comes to the entrance of Kent Lake Park. She has found the correct entrance and goes to the parking lot by the east boat launch. Andrea finds Angela's car and parks next to it. Vickie and Kim are already there. Andrea joins them.

"How is your training going?" Angela asks the ladies.

"Going very well," replies Andrea.

"I am doing great!" replies Vickie.

"I have managed to squeeze my training in with my busy work schedule," Kim replies.

Doree, Sharon and Denese all arrive in the same vehicle and then Karin drives in. Everyone gathers around by Angela's car.

"We are going to head over to the trail and take it to the left. This will give us a nice hilly terrain and we'll end up going along by the water. It'll be great scenery. We will practice our trail etiquette just as we have on the other trails. Let's all head out now," instructs Angela.

They all walk from the parking lot to the trail and go left. The trail is twists and turns at this point but remains level. As the ladies head into the trees the trail descends with a nice downward slope. The road into the park is next to them. The trail goes uphill and winds between the highway and the lake.

As the walkers continue the trail splits into two paths, one goes under the highway the other goes across a bridge. Angela instructs, "Vickie and Andrea, go across the bridge."

A short distance after the bridge the trail follows the water's edge where there are fishing docks off the trail. The ladies follow the trail to the entrance of the west boat launch.

When they turn around at the entrance they go around the outside of the playground, just for fun.

"This park is very scenic. I like the change from training in the downtown areas," says Kim.

"I agree with you," replies Doree.

"It is a lot quieter out here too," adds Andrea.

Denese adds, "I am actually enjoying the challenging and rolling hills."

"My calves are really feeling it," Karin adds in.

Angela says to the group, "I am glad to hear you ladies like this area. It'll be a great place to meet up and walk after the race."

They get to the first fishing dock and they all go out on it and then Angela has them all gather close together and takes a selfie of the group.

Continuing along the trail there are many bikers that pass them. Many times, Vickie or Andrea will shout out "bikes up" and Andrea and Karin at the back will shout out "bikes back."

They make their way to the bridge. Here they stop in the middle, gather closely together and take another selfie. The easy part of the trail was behind them, ahead of them is the hilly trail.

The group makes it back by the east boat dock. They take the ramp down to the dock area and then walk back up to the trail and continue their walk to the beach area. Angela walks to the front of the group and then leads them across the sandy beach. A short time later, they return to the parking lot and Angela's car.

Denese goes to her car and gets the treats. She opens the cooler that contains fruit snacks and juice boxes.

Angela says to the group, "you ladies have done a great job of keeping up with your homework. It shows in your walking during our group walks. I have seen great improvement over the last few weeks. We have completed 7 weeks which means we are down to 3 weeks before the race. Be sure to get your race clothes figured out this weekend including your shoes. Have you figured out what is good for you for breakfast before the race? You have only 3 more Saturdays to plan your pre-race morning. The morning of the race we will meet at the grocery store's parking lot by University at 6 am and then cross the road to the start line. Before we cross the road we will use the pharmacy's restrooms. Any questions?"

"No" they all reply.

"Ok, next week we will be meeting at Oakland State University, parking deck D. Doree will be bringing the goodies. Everyone have a safe drive home and I'll see you next week." Angela tells them.

"See you next week," everyone replies.

Everyone goes to their vehicles and heads out of the park. Andrea gets in her truck and drives to her ex's house to get the boys. She grabs a Phyzix Zero out of her personal cooler on the passenger seat.

Andrea finally arrives at Michael's house. Andrea gets out of her truck and goes up to the front door and rings the doorbell. Carson comes running to the door with Cooper right behind him. Carson opens the door, Andrea walks in and gives both boys a hug and kiss.

She says to Michael, "thanks for watching them on Thursdays for me. It's been really nice to train with my walking group."

"You're welcome." replies Michael.

"Time to go home boys, get your stuff." Andrea tells the boys. They grab their stuff, get their shoes on and then give their dad a big hug.

"Good bye dad!" the boys tell him. Andrea and the boys get into her truck and drive off towards home.

They arrive home, and she parks in the garage. Andrea and the boys get out of the truck and go inside.

Andrea sets her stuff down on the dining room table. The boys run up to their room and get their pajamas on. She follows them up the stairs and goes to her room.

After getting her pajamas on she goes into the boys' room, sits down next to Cooper on his bed and picks up a book off of their book shelf between their beds.

"How about a bedtime story?" she asks.

"Yeah!" both boys reply.

Carson jumps over onto Cooper's bed so that he can see the book. The boys both help with turning the pages.

"The end," Andrea says as she finishes the book.

Carson goes back over to his bed and gets under his blankets. Cooper slides under his blankets. She gives them both a hug and kiss.

"Good night boys."

"Good night mom!"

Chapter 16: Tree House Fun

The main entrance features a dark brown wood sign that says "Merkley Nature Preserve" and has green trees and a blue river on it. There is a long winding driveway that is lined with a variety of trees on the way to the parking lot. Andrea rolls down her window, so they can smell the flowers and listen to the gravel under the tires as they drive back to the parking lot. Andrea parks her truck close to the dark wood framed information board.

"Hey boys, ready to go walking?" asks Andrea.

"Yeah!" the boys holler.

The boys hop down out of the truck and stand by the information board. Carson spots the sign for the tree house off to the left. "Mom! Look! The tree house!" he says and points at the sign.

"Ok, let's go to the tree house boys," Andrea says and takes their hands as they walk towards the sign for the tree house. On the sign is a picture of the tree house and the hours it is open. They follow the paved pathway to the ramp of the tree house. This tree house is barrier free and has a long winding ramp up to the door. At the entrance to the ramp the boys let go of Andrea's hands and run up the ramp to the door where there are metal sculptures of a bear and a fox.

"Come on in," says the park guide, who is sitting inside the tree house.

As they enter the tree house Cooper looks up and says, "Cool! A Frog!" There's a large frog head on the wall right above a chalkboard. They look around and see a tree that is coming up through the floor in one spot and exiting through the roof in two spots. On the tree is a wasps' nest that is about the size of the boy's heads. There are benches along the outer walls and windows above them.

There's a door next to the chalkboard that leads out to a balcony. Andrea takes the boys hands and says, "we can go out there, but no goofing around."

Out on the balcony they look down into the swampy area that still has water in it from recent rains. Off to the left is Kearsley Creek where there are a couple of Canadian geese that are swimming by. The one goose is honking and honking, after a few minutes the other goose responds, and they swim off up the creek.

They go back inside, and the boys sit down on the floor and Andrea sits on a bench to listen while the park guide reads a book on tree creatures.

"The end," says the park guide and everyone claps.

Everyone gets up and some go out on the balcony while others leave. Andrea and the boys leave the tree house and take the stairs down to the tic-tac-toe tree stumps. There is a sign that says to play tic-tac-toe you need to pick up nature things. The boys pick up some rocks and twigs. Carson wins the first game and Cooper wins the second game.

"Alright boys let's go walk over by the pond and see if we can see any turtles," Andrea says.

"Ok," the boys reply.

They follow the trail back towards the parking lot and walk to the nature center building. Andrea and the boys walk towards the dirt trail behind the nature center building. They see a sign that says Quiet Area. Andrea leads them to the right where the path goes between two ponds. They can peak through the tall grass and see the pond on the right has slimy pea green water. They stand still and listen to the bull frogs making raspy, throaty, croaking noises.

Andrea and the boys continue along the path. The path splits and they take the path to the left. The boys get to the lookout tower, stop and look out onto the pond where there is a Canadian goose swimming close to the shoreline. Andrea taps them on the shoulders, puts her finger to her lips and points to the stairs of the lookout tower. They all tip toe to the stairs and go up without making any noise.

At the top of the tower the boys get up on the bench seats to look over the sides. Carson sees the Canadian goose walking up the bank of the pond and it stops in the middle of the path to peck at the grass. Carson looks back at Cooper and motions for him to come over next to him. Cooper quietly moves next to Carson. The goose walks under the lookout tower.

Cooper gets down, tip toes down the stairs and turns around to look through the steps at the goose. The goose stays on the opposite side of the lookout tower and stops to look at Cooper. It then walks towards the pond and Cooper peeks around the side of the stairs to see the goose looking back at him. The goose turns away, walks down the bank and into the pond.

Andrea and Carson join Cooper at the bottom of the stairs. They continue their walk around the pond and discover dozens of orange carp swimming around the water covered dock. To the right of the dock there is a painted turtle on a log.

Carson turns around and through the trees he sees a path leading to a couple of logs being held with guide wires. He tugs on Andrea's hand and points to what he sees. She turns to see the bridge posts. Taking both boys by the hand Andrea walks with them to the bridge. It's a suspension bridge.

Carson goes first onto the wooden planks and they move as he steps on them. Cooper joins him and then Andrea says to them, "boys, turn this way so I can take a picture." They turn to her and smile. After taking the picture she joins them on the bridge. They all jump up and down and the bridge goes up and down with their movements.

Cooper says, "let's race across the bridge." They all go to the end of the bridge where Carson and Cooper stand next to each other.

"Ready? Set? Go!" says Andrea and the boys are off across the bridge.

Cooper nudges out Carson for the win. "I win!" exclaims Cooper.

Catching up to the boys Andrea says, "let's go see what else is on the path." She takes their hands and they walk further along the path going up the hill back to the "Quiet Area" sign.

Walking across the parking area they go down a path that leads to another pond. A brown wooden arched gateway leads to the pond. In the center of the pond is an island with a tree. There is a Canadian goose on the island pecking away at the grass. To the left of the island is a fallen tree branch in the water with a large painted turtle basking in the heat from the sun.

When they turn around, they see another Canadian goose laying in the shade under a tree and it appears to be sleeping with its beak tucked into its feathers. Tiptoeing through the grass they quietly step back onto the path and head to the truck.

At the truck Andrea gets the cooler out and they walk over to the picnic table area for lunch. "Here's an extra crunchy peanut butter sandwich for Carson and a strawberry jelly sandwich for Cooper."

"Yeah!" both boys reply.

"Here's a bag of corn chips for us all to share," she puts the bag on the table in between the boys. Andrea sits down across the table from them with her apple cider jelly and extra crunchy peanut butter sandwich.

They finish their lunch, put their wrappers in the trash can and take their cooler to the truck. They get in their seats. She backs out of her parking space to drive down the winding driveway to head for home.

Chapter 17: Week 8

It is a warm sunny Thursday afternoon and Andrea is outside on the front porch while Carson and Cooper are playing in the driveway. Michael drives up and parks his truck across the end of the driveway. The boys put their stuff in the garage and run to give their dad a hug as he walks up the driveway.

"Hey boys let's go get some dinner."

"YEAH!!!" the boys holler.

They give Andrea a hug and kiss good bye and head out for dinner with their dad.

Andrea goes inside to get her stuff for walking. Then she gets in her truck and drives to Oakland State University. The parking deck that she needs to park in is in the middle of campus, so she has a bit of a drive once she gets on campus. The campus is nice and hilly. She gets to the parking deck and goes round and round and round until she gets to the top deck. She spots Angela's car and Andrea pulls into a parking spot next to Angela. She removes her walking gear from her and sets it close to Angela's car.

"Hi!" Andrea says to Angela.

"Hi! How's it going?" Angela replies.

"It's going great."

"Wonderful."

Vickie arrives and pulls into a spot next to Andrea. She joins Andrea and Angela.

"Hi ladies!" Vickie says.

"Hi!" they reply.

"How's it going?" Angela asks Vickie.

"Great. I've been walking everywhere around town. I take my backpack with me for small shopping trips. It's nice having everything so close to home.

Slowly everyone arrives. Angela says to her group of ladies, "today we are going to have a very different workout. We are going to do a few hills on the sidewalk right out front here and then we'll walk around campus. It'll be a good workout. We'll end with our goodies back here that Doree brought tonight. Let's get walking!"

The ladies walk out of the parking lot from the top deck where they are in the middle of a hill. They walk down the hill to the base, which is right before the entrance to the parking deck. "We are going to do walking sprints up the hill. Go as fast as you can but remain walking. We will go to the stop sign up ahead. Ready?" Angela asks.

"Ready!" the group replies.

"Let's go!" Angela shouts. The ladies takeoff up the hill with Vickie in the lead and Andrea hot on her heels. Following closely behind are Kim, Denese, Doree, Sharon and Karin with Angela bringing up the back of the group.

"Ok ladies, we are now going to go back down the hill and come back up. Remember, only walking, no running." They all go down the hill to the bottom. At the bottom they all wait for everyone to gather before going up the hill. The ladies head up the hill with Andrea in the lead this time followed very closely by Vickie then Kim, Sharon, Doree, Denese, Karin and Angela.

"We are done with these hills, for now. Let's go to our next challenge." Angela says to the group. They walk across the sidewalk that leads to the Recreation Center and as they reach the sidewalk next to Recreation Center Angela informs the group, "we are going to walk down the hill and come back up the hill."

Everyone walks down the hill and gathers at the bottom. "When we go up the hill be careful with your footing. We want to be quick but not injured," Angela informs the group.

Next, they all sprint up the hill. This hill has room for the group to run side by side. Angela notes their pace to be near equal. As they all reach the sidewalk they take a drink from their water bottles. Angela compliments them, "you ladies did a great job of getting up that hill!"

"Follow me." Angela says and leads the group around the front of the Recreation Center to the front steps of the arena.

"Now we are going to go up and down these stairs in a figure eight. So, we will start out going down this side of the stairs, up the other side of the wall, down the last section and then up the middle section and so forth."

Angela leads the group down the stairs and they are all in a single file line going down and then up the stairs. This goes on for about 10 minutes and they end at the top of the stairs. "All right! We'll go down the ramp and around the building to the right. Let's go!" she encourages.

Angela has Vickie and Andrea lead the group. They go down the ramp and as they go around the building to the right they form a single file line. As Vickie gets to the parking lot she leads the ladies down the aisle and then to the left and to the right where they get to a wood staircase leading down to the softball fields. Angela takes the lead and says, "we'll go down these stairs, back up the stairs and we'll repeat it one time."

The stairs are in a group of trees and you can hear the squirrels playing in the tree tops above. As they are going down the stairs off to the left at the bottom, a couple of deer are walking by, not bothered by our presence as we come down the stairs. They get to the bottom of the stairs and turn around and go back up the stairs, they do it once again and gather at the top of the stairs.

"Ok, we are going to go back down the stairs one more time and then up the hill that we went up earlier. This will take us back to the parking deck. We will do one more hill and then back to our vehicles. Let's go!" Angela instructs them. The group heads down the stairs with Kim and Denese leading the way this time. They walk across the grass until they are near the south end of the Recreation Center and then hike up the hill.

At the top of the hill they take a drink from their water bottles before continuing to their last hill. The sidewalk is nice and empty allowing the walkers to walk 2 by 2. Sharon and Doree lead the way across the sidewalk and down the hill next to the parking deck. They get to the bottom of the hill and Angela says, "this is our last hill. When we get to the sidewalk from the parking deck we will follow it to our vehicles. We'll be done walking for this week. Everyone ready!"

"YES!" the group replies. Andrea and Vickie lead the group up the hill and back to their vehicles.

They arrive at their vehicles and gather around Angela's car. Doree stops at her car and gets the cooler full of goodies, which are sliced strawberries, seedless green grapes and bottles of water. She puts the cooler in the back of Angela's opened car.

Angela informs her group, "Excellent job tonight ladies! You will be sore tomorrow and/or Saturday. Next week will be our last walk together prior to the race. We will meet at the grocery store's parking lot by University. Our walk is only going to be 35 minutes and Sharon will be bringing our goodies. The expo will take place on Saturday, Sunday, Monday and Tuesday. There is no packet pick up the morning of the race. I will send you an email that contains the exact expo times. When you know you are going let everyone know and then some of you can meet up and go through the expo together. I advise taking all the free samples you want, however don't eat or drink anything new prior to the race. There will be a lot of deals at the expo, buy what you want, but don't wear anything new to the race. This is a 5K and to some it may seem overly cautious for a short race. However, if you get in the habit of doing these things for the short races it will be easier to do when you are training and getting ready for longer races. I'll see everyone next week."

Everyone goes to their vehicles and leaves for the evening. Andrea drives home because Michael is dropping the boys off after they get done eating.

Chapter 18: Finally to the Gym

"Good morning!" says Amy as Andrea walks through the door at Fitness for Life gym.

"Good morning! I have a 5-day pass from the Oakland Training Program," replies Andrea.

"Great, let me get Jessie for you," grabbing the iPad, bringing up the guest sign-in screen, Amy turns the iPad to Andrea, "please fill this out." "Jessie, you have a guest from the Oakland Training Program," Amy says over the walkie talkies.

"I'll be right there," replies Jessie.

Andrea turns the iPad back to Amy, "ok, Jessie will be right up. You can have a seat in our lobby area right on the other side of the wall," says Amy. Andrea walks over and has a seat on the couch in the lobby.

A few moments later Jessie walks up to Andrea, "Hi! I am Jessie and I understand that you are from the Oakland Training Program. Welcome. Let me give you a tour of the facility and then I will have you see Angela."

"Hi! Nice to meet you Jessie. Angela is my group leader in the training program," Andrea replies and stands up to shake Jessie's hand.

"Great," pointing and moving towards the spa, "over here is our spa. They offer services on nails, hair and skin along with massage." Turning to the window next to the spa, "this is our indoor pool area and through those doors at the other side is our outdoor pool and patio. We'll go in there shortly. In here is the family locker room for members with children of the opposite sex. Do you have children?"

"Yes, I have two boys, they are 5 years old," replies Andrea.

"What are their names?" she asks.

"Carson and Cooper," Andrea says. Jessie then motions for them to walk through the lobby area and continue through the hallway.

"This is our member services desk, where you can get your questions answered about your membership if you join us," pointing to the left next to the lobby. "Over here is our cafe. They have wonderful smoothies and great food. You'll want to check out the specials when you are here. Along this wall are our supplements and then quick items. On the left here are the offices of our account managers. This one is mine. We'll come back here when you're done today. Anytime you have any questions, just let me know."

They continue to the end of the hall, "on the left is our member activities desk where you can find out about camps and special activities going on for members. Next is the area of our chiropractor and physical therapist. Over here to the right, you can go to the next level, using either by the stairs or the elevator. In front of us is one of our gyms. We have two gyms side by side and as we look inside the gym you'll see the rock climbing wall. Have you ever been rock climbing?" Jessie asks.

"No, I haven't but I would love to try it some time," Andrea replies as she looks into the gym.

"This would be the perfect place to try it. Let's continue, the next door goes to both gyms. On the left, we have the men's locker room, the towel desk and the women's locker room. We'll go through there in just a few minutes. Let's go in this door to see what else is in the gym," Jessie points out. "Quite often the kids camps come in here and have a bounce house set up or they play games. Here we have a spinning class where you can reserve your bike on-line ahead of time. Let's peek into the kids' area," she suggests as they leave the gym area.

"The child care area offers a full tour with all the details. When you bring the boys with you a tour will be available. The child care is included with membership," Jessie tells her. "Let's continue on and go through the women's locker room," says Jessie while directing her to the entry of the women's locker room. "Here we have a nice lounge area with a television and a remote for your convenience. Your membership card gives you access to the locker and a locker key. A safety pin is attached to the key for your convenience. We have hair dryers, along with hand lotion. There is a steam room in each locker room. This interesting contraption here is a dryer for your swimsuit. You put your suit in and hold down the lid. Down here we have the showers and in each shower is a soap dispenser. Let's go out into the pool area," Jessie motions for them to walk through the shower area.

"Do you and the boys like to swim?" Jessie asks.

"Yes, we do. We haven't been in a while though. There is a pool at our townhouse complex, but it's usually really crowded and no life guard on duty," Andrea replies.

"This is our lap pool, which is primarily for adults. On occasion we may have swim lessons for kids in there, but that's generally only when we are doing maintenance on our leisure pool. That's the leisure pool over there where there is zero entry. It also has slides and a fountain. Over here are our wonderful 12-person hot tubs. The kids are too young to go in there, but you can enjoy them. Right here is our sauna. Let's go outside. This area is open from sunrise to sunset for adults and then we have family swim starting at 10 am and the slides and fountains are on starting at 11. Over here it is the zero entry. Being that they are 5, you will need to have them take a swim test or you will have to remain in the water with them. Do you have any questions so far?" Jessie asks.

"Not so far. I am looking forward to meeting with Angela and getting in a good workout. I will probably use the gym primarily when the boys are at their dad's," replies Andrea.

"Ok, well, let's go upstairs and meet with Angela then," Jessie tells her. They go through the family locker room and down the hallway to go up the stairs to the personal training desk. "Is this your first year with the training program?" asks Jessie.

"Yes, it is. I saw a commercial for it and decided to go for it. So far, I have really enjoyed training with the group. Angela and the rest of my group has been great," Andrea tells her.

"Hi Angela!" says Jessie as they approach the personal training desk where Angela is at with a couple of trainers. "I have Andrea here. I understand that she is in your walking group."

"Hi Jessie and Andrea," replies Angela. "I'll take Andrea and show her around up here. Thanks Jessie."

"You are in great hands Andrea. When you are done up here, stop by my office. Thanks Angela," says Jessie.

"Ok Andrea, let me show what we have going on here. We'll do the tour, then we'll get your stats and finally what you've been waiting for, a workout," Angela explains.

"Sounds good. I got a large tour of the first floor. Lots to do just down there," Andrea replies.

"Yes, this is a pretty large facility with a variety of stuff to do for everyone. We'll start right over here. This is our stretching area. We have mats, exercise balls, foam rollers and stretching chairs. The windows let you see what's going on in the gym below. Lots of basketball games are played down there. The personal training desk, which is right where I was at when you guys came upstairs, is where you can go to find a trainer and ask any questions. They can help you with equipment and anything else you need. The room on the right is a group fitness studio. The class schedule is on-line and on the door. Next, we have our cardio equipment. This includes ellipticals, treadmills, bikes, and stair climbers. We also have tv's that you can watch while working out. On our cardio equipment you can bring up

Netflix and other internet-based videos. There's a headphone jack or you can use blue-tooth," Angela informs her.

"That's awesome! I love Netflix," replies Andrea.

"Now, let's go over here. This is our weight machine area. Each row focuses on a different part of the body. So, you have a row for abdominals, arms, chest, shoulders, back, and legs. Each machine has instructions right on them showing you how to use it. You can reference the videos that are linked to the QR code that is on the machine. A trainer is always available to assist you, too. This way you will know how to properly use the machines," says Angela.

Walking by the machines they go by another room. "This is our yoga studio. The schedule is also on-line or on the door. Normally they have the room a bit dark with fireless candles on. It's a sound proof room so that there is no disturbance from the other room. They do ask that no one comes into the room more than 5 minutes late due to disturbing the rest of the class. We'll continue around this corner up here," Angela points the way.

"I haven't tried yoga before. I will have to give that a try. What other classes do you have here?" questions Andrea.

"We have Zumba, dance jam, cardio kickboxing, TCX, which is strength training, cardio and high intensity, and a lot more classes. We can go over a schedule and see what you'd like to try, or you can go on the website and browse at your leisure," answers Angela. "Over here we have more treadmills, mats, foam rollers and exercise balls. Next, we have the free weight area. Let me know if you would like any assistance with doing free weights."

"I think I will stick to the weight machines. I am not a fan of the free weights," Andrea replies.

"In this corner is our Pilates studio. You can get one class for free and after that you can buy a package of classes. This sums up the tour of this area. Let's go over to get your weight and body stats. We will review it and then you get a copy of it each time we weigh you in so that you can see your progress. Do you have any questions so far?"

"How often do we weigh in? What other stats do you go over?" questions Andrea.

"We will weigh you today and then as often as you like. That can be once a month, one a quarter, whenever you like. I'll show you what all it prints out. It's amazing. Take your shoes and socks off, step up on the scale and hold the handles loosely down by your sides but not touching your sides," instructs Angela. "We wait until it shows complete on the screen and then you can step off."

Andrea steps off the scale and puts her shoes and socks back on. The printer spits out her results.

"Ok, let me explain what the scale shows us. This shows your weight along with total body water, lean body mass and body measurements. It does give your BMI, which I don't use because with athletes it does not accurately categorize them. We do want to watch the percent of body fat and work towards getting that lower," Angela informs her.

"Now that we have completed all that, let's get you started out on the elliptical. Have you been on an elliptical before?" asks Angela.

"Yes, I have," replies Andrea.

"Ok, we will have you do the elliptical for 30 minutes. After the 30 minutes we will go over to the stretching area and do the stretches that I had given you previously. When you are done with the stretches we can go over a schedule of exercises for your other 4 days of free trial here. At the end of your last free day we will sit down and talk with Jessie about what she can do for you for membership pricing," says Angela.

"Sounds good to me," Andrea says and gets on the elliptical. She sets the exercise program to cardio for 30 minutes and then puts on Netflix, signs in and selects NCIS.

Thirty minutes later the elliptical changes into a 10-minute cool down. Angela walks over to Andrea, "So, how do you feel?"

"It went by pretty quickly and I feel great, of course I haven't stepped off it yet. So, we shall see," Andrea chuckles.

The elliptical comes to an end and Andrea gets off and takes the cleaner from Angela. "This cleaner and towels are right over by the desk and at various areas around the equipment. Always clean off the equipment when you are done. For the elliptical clean off the handles and anywhere you touch, such as the screen and the water bottle holder. There are receptacles around the gym for used towels."

Walking over to the stretching area, "here's a mat and let's stretch right here. What are your thoughts so far about the gym?" Angela asks while they are stretching.

"So far, I like it all. I am impressed with what all is here. I can see myself working out here while the boys are at their dad's. Maybe in time, once I get a good routine down I'll bring them along, but right now I like it for me," she responds.

"I am trying to get everyone in my group to at least try the gym out once. I highly recommend checking the schedule out for the yoga classes. They will pair very well with your cardio and group workouts."

"We can put it in my schedule of workouts. The boys go to their dad's on the weekends. I can also get him to watch them during the week.

"Now that we have the stretching done let's go sit up to the desk and see what we can do about your 4 days," Angela says as they clean the mats and put them away.

Sitting at the desk, Andrea gets her phone out with her schedule on it. Angela asks, "which days do you want to come? You mentioned the weekends. You have one more weekend before the race and I see that we have a yoga class at 10 am. Will that work for you?"

"Yes, let me add that in. What do I bring to yoga class?" Andrea replies.

"Just yourself unless you happen to have your own yoga mat. They have them there. Oh yeah, you may want to bring a bottle of water. We'll put the yoga class again on your schedule for the Saturday after the race and then pick a day after that to get on the elliptical."

"How about on Wednesday at 6 pm? Will you be here?" asks Andrea.

"I will be here and after you get done with your workout we'll talk with Jessie. Right now, though, let's go downstairs and see Jessie. For your next visit you can bring a change of clothes or change after you get here. Feel free to use the locker room."

They walk down the stairs to Jessie's office. "Hey Jessie, we are done with her workout and she'll be back next week for yoga class," Angela says.

"Sounds good. Andrea it was great to meet you and feel free to ask any questions when you are here. Here's my card and you can email me as well. Enjoy your next 4 visits and we'll talk more on your last visit," Jessie shakes Andrea's hand.

Angela walks Andrea to the front, "glad you came, and I'll see you on Thursday."

"Thanks. See you Thursday."

Andrea heads to her truck.

Chapter 19: Week 9

Andrea is sitting in the kitchen and thinking to herself *it is incredible that tonight is the final night of training before the race. I am excited and sad all at the same time. I have made some great friends and have enjoyed meeting with them weekly.*

Carson and Cooper go running to the front door because their dad is in the driveway. Michael parks his truck and walks up to the door. The boys open the door and Michael comes inside. "Alright boys let me in the door. We will have some pizza and watch tv." Michael tells the boys.

"Carson and Cooper, I am going to be leaving shortly. You guys be good for your dad." Andrea says while putting her shoes on. The boys give her a hug and kiss goodbye. She goes out to her truck and drives to her group meet-up location.

Vickie and Andrea are the first ones at the location. They get out of their vehicles.

"Hi!" Vickie says.

"Hi! How's it going?" Andrea replies.

"Great. I've been doing all of my homework and the exercises every day."

"Awesome! The exercises really help."

Angela drives up and then the rest of the group joins them.

"Good evening ladies! Tonight, is our last group walk before the race. We are going to do the race route and then we will come back here for goodies that Sharon brought. Let's go!" Angela instructed the group.

The group goes across the road at the traffic light. "We are going to start part way into the course so that we aren't doubling up tonight. We will go to the start/finish line before we are done tonight. First, we are going to continue down to the entrance." Angela instructs her group.

The group walks 2 by 2 down the sidewalk and gets to the university entrance and turns right. Vickie and Andrea lead the group a short distance and then they turn left to go towards the Black Forest Hall. This is a nice winding road that goes downhill into the entry area by the garages of Black Forest Hall. They walk across the brick and get to the roundabout and turn right and then turn right, again, onto the small bridge that is canopied by trees. There are many birds hidden in the trees chirping as they walk by.

Immediately past the trees they walk by a white fence and turn to the left where the road leads to the soccer fields. The group comes to a challenging hill that goes to the right. Vickie and Andrea are still at the front of the group and Angela and Karin are bringing up the back of the group. The group is close together in pace. The sun is shining brightly and heating the asphalt as they continue their training walk.

At the top of the hill Angela says, "Let's stop and take a water break. Along the race route there will be water stops. With this being a 5K, there will be only one. I highly recommend that you carry water with you. It's going to be a hot one, so make sure that you also have electrolytes."

After a few minutes, "alright, let's get back moving." Angela takes the lead along with Andrea.

They go to the right where they head alongside some soccer fields and towards the on-campus housing. The next intersection they get to, they cross over and go down the stairs and are walking along the on-campus housing. The road on the other side of the housing is getting busy and the traffic is noisy.

Once they get to the road that comes in from the main road they wait for traffic to clear and then cross. The path continues alongside the on-campus road. Angela cautions the walkers to be aware of the vehicles passing by so near to the path. This path leads to the entrance of Black Forest Hall where the start/finish line is.

"Ladies, this is where we will start and finish. There will be tents here on the left for the post-race goodies and lots of port-a-johns. We will head back to our vehicles now. We are a short distance away." Angela informs the group. They take the path along the main road lined with trees. They head to the traffic light, wait for the crossing signal, and safely return to their vehicles.

Sharon gets the goodies out of her vehicle and puts them in the back end of Angela's car. Sharon brought mini-cupcakes for celebrating their great training plus some small bottles of chocolate milk. It is a special treat night.

Angela instructs them, "Now that we have completed the race route you ladies are all ready for the race. We will meet here at 6:00 am, race day. Yes, this seems early, but due to road closures it's easier for us to be here early. Plus, we can cheer on those going out for races ahead of ours. Before the race day you will need to go to the race expo. Make sure that you email me when you will be going to the expo so that I can get the list out to everyone. It's been great fun training with you ladies. Have a great evening and see you at the expo and/or race morning here."

"I am planning on going to the expo on Sunday," says Vickie.

"Me too," chimes in Kim.

"I'll be there on Sunday also," says Denese.

"I'll check and see, but I think that I can make it then also," Andrea adds.

Karin says, "I am going on Monday."

"Monday works for me," says Doree.

"I'll see Kim, Denese and Andrea on Sunday and Karin and Doree race morning. Which are you going to Angela?" inquires Vickie.

"Sunday looks like it'll work for me."

The ladies go to their vehicles. Andrea gets into her truck and drives home. She has a few miles to drive home. When she arrives home she pulls her truck into the garage.

Andrea goes into her townhouse, "Carson and Cooper, I am home!!!"

The boys come running up to her from the living room and give her a hug. She takes her shoes off and goes into the living room.

"How were the boys?" she asks Michael. "They were really good. We had pizza and the boys watched Scooby Doo," he replies.

"Glad to hear it." She says.

"Well boys, time for me to go and you guys to get ready for bed." Michael says to the boys. They give him a hug and kiss and then head upstairs to get ready for bed.

Michael leaves and Andrea heads upstairs to get on her pajamas. She tucks Cooper and Carson into bed and then lays in bed reading her book.

Chapter 20: Race Expo

Andrea looks once again at the email Angela sent out with the times that everyone is going to be at the expo. She sees that Vickie and Angela are going to be there at 2:00 pm and she looks at her fitness watch to see what time it is. Yes, almost time for her to go. Andrea thinks to herself *I am really excited about going to my first expo and the great thing is I get to do it with my group.*

It is time to go, Andrea gets her shoes on and gets into her truck. She drives over to the University to meet everyone. Parking is a bit of a challenge, even though it is a Sunday; so many people are there for the expo. After a few minutes she finds a parking spot and walks over to the Recreation Center. The expo is downstairs on the basketball courts and she walks down the stairs. Andrea finds Vickie and Angela and as she is walking up to them Kim and Denese walk up.

Angela advises them, "We are going to walk through and get our bib number and goodie bag first and then we will go through the vendors. Again, I advise that you do not drink or eat anything new. Clothing that you purchase today should not be worn the morning of the race. Let's go get our stuff ladies."

"Let's go!" they all shout.

The ladies walk through the maze of vendors to get to where the list of race participants are posted on a wall. They each find their name and bib number on the long list. Andrea's number is 83070. They get into the 5K line and pick up their bib number. The 5K walk line isn't nearly as long as the half marathon line.

Vickie says, "it doesn't really matter how long the lines are because we get to enjoy each other's company."

"Once we get our bib number and shirt we'll meet over at the Oakland Races table." Angela says to the group.

Andrea finally gets her bib number, goodie bag and t-shirt and goes over to the table. She and Vickie wait for the rest of the group. They are looking at all the Oakland races merchandise.

Andrea says, "I am getting a mug and a 5K sticker."

Vickie comments, "I'll get a 5K sticker as well."

The rest of the group joins them.

"I like the mugs. I'll take one," says Denese.

"I am going to be different and get a jacket," Kim adds in.

Angela says to Jenni, the lady working the table for the Oakland Races, "I do believe I get a mug for being a group leader and I would also like a hat."

"Yes, you do get a mug. Thanks for being a group leader. Here's your hat," Jenni replies.

They all walk over to the free massage booth. Stephania says, "hi ladies, who would like a massage?"

Andrea speaks up first, "I will. This will be my first ever chair massage."

As she is sitting there she thinks to herself *I need to figure out how to work massages into my schedule and budget.*

With six chairs they all get massages at the same time.

After their massages the ladies walk along to the booth for the Detroit races which has race fliers for the marathon and the Thanksgiving race. Andrea and Vickie pick up a flier for the Thanksgiving race.

"I could do this." says Andrea.

Vickie replies "Yes, you can, and I can do it with you."

The group continue along to a booth with all kinds of running and walking jewelry. There are charms, beads, pendant, rings, bracelets, necklaces and earrings.

Andrea finds a silver snake chain necklace, "I like this, and I will also get these the rectangular charm that says "Keep Moving" on one side and "Don't Stop" on the reverse side, the running shoe charm, the bead that says WALK on it, the circular 5K charm and three charm spacers."

Vickie says, "I will get the pink Swarovski round faceted crystal charm that is accented with a small sterling silver daisy."

Angela reminds the group again, "I highly recommend not taking samples of something you have never tried before. You don't know how your body will react to it," as they pass by a booth that is handing out samples of some new energy red energy drink in small bathroom size paper cups.

The booth right after it is a local running store and the ladies walk around looking at all the deals on sports bras, running shorts, tank tops, jelly beans, Gu, and various other running and walking accessories.

The next booth is for the local parks system and Andrea picks up all the maps that they have available. She thinks to herself *I like finding some new places to take the boys where I can walk, and they can ride their bikes.*

A local grocery store has the next booth that the ladies go to and they all pick up bottles of water and chewy granola bars. There are also 3" x 5" cards with recipes on the table for them to pick up, too. Andrea takes one of each of the recipes.

There are quite a few booths with samples of various drinks and snacks, which the ladies disregard. They are back at the start of the expo, Angela says, "is there any booth that anyone wants to go back to?"

"No" everyone responds.

"Alright, everyone that wants to join me, I am going to the Coney Island over on Livernois. We can talk about any of your concerns about the race," Angela invites the group.

Andrea says, "I'll go."

Vickie responds, "I'm game and it's right near home for me."

Kim and Denese look at each other and then say, "we'll meet you over there."

The ladies all go to their vehicles and drive over to the Coney Island. The hostess says, "welcome, how many?"

"Five, can we have a round table?" Angela replies.

Cindi, the waitress brings them all red plastic glasses of ice water, "are you ready to order?"

"Yes, I will have two coney dogs with no onions or mustard plus fries," says Andrea.

Vickie orders, "I will have a Greek salad."

Kim says, "I will have a chicken gyro sandwich with rice."

Denese orders, "I will have a bacon, lettuce and tomato sandwich with fries."

Lastly, Angela says, "I will have a chicken Caesar wrap."

"Thank you, I will get these orders in," says Cindi and she walks away towards the kitchen.

"Now that we have all of food ordered I wanted to ask you ladies if you have any questions about the race coming up on Wednesday." Angela says to the group.

"How will we line up for the race?" asks Andrea.

"When it's time for us to line up we will go to the color of the flag that matches our bib color. Once in that corral we will go towards the back of it." Angela replies.

"Will there be bathrooms at the start/finish line?" asks Vickie.

Angela replies, "yes there will be lots of port-a-johns around the start/finish line. There will be a row on each side of the sponsor tent."

Denese asks, "what will be available to eat after the race, post race goodie wise?"

"There will be fruit and salty snacks in the finish line area such as bananas, apples and various flavors of chips. Plus there will be water in the finish line area. In the post race celebration tent there will be a cash bar. On your race bib there are two tear off tickets at the bottom, one is for beer or pop and the other is for pizza. There are also a few local restaurants that will have food available for purchase. So, lots to eat and drink available after the race. Be sure to put some cash in a baggy in your waist pack," Angela informs them.

Their food arrives, and the ladies are busy eating and not talking. After they are done eating the waitress comes and takes away all the dishes. "Any more questions?" asks Angela.

"Will there be a place for my boys to see me start and finish?" inquires Andrea.

"Yes, there will be a set of bleachers right by the start/finish line that they can sit on. It's near where we will be standing to cheer on the runners and walkers that go out ahead of us." replies Angela.

She then asks, "Anything else?" No one says anything, but they all shake their heads no.

"Ok, so we will meet at 6:00 am in the parking lot of the grocery store that is facing University. After everyone arrives we will walk over to the pharmacy and use their restrooms before we cross the road and walk over to the start/finish area. We are arriving early because they shut down many of the roads that would lead us to great parking a few minutes before the start of the half marathon. After the 10K race goes out we will walk to our corral for the 5K. We will stay together as a group during the race, actually I think our paces will keep us all pretty close together anyway. After the race we will go into the post race celebration tent to get our free food and beverage and any other food and beverages we want." Angela informs the group.

Cindi brings their individual bills. The ladies all get up, walk over to the cash register, check out and go to their vehicles.

Andrea gets into her truck and drives home. Michael has the boys for a few more hours, so she goes in her townhouse and goes through her stretches in front of the tv.

Chapter 21: Race Prep

It's the day before the race and Andrea is just waking up to the sun peeking through her window blinds. The townhouse is so quiet with the boys gone to their dad's. She gets up, gets dressed and goes downstairs to the kitchen for breakfast.

What to eat for breakfast? Angela thinks to herself. She fixes a bowl of oatmeal with raisins, brown sugar and maple syrup along with a glass of low-acid, pulp-free orange juice. Sitting down to eat breakfast Andrea has her laptop open and she is browsing through her email.

There's an email from Angela, "Good morning walkers! It's been a great training season and you are ready to take on this race. I want to make sure that you are ready for race morning. Here's a list of things you will want to do today to make tomorrow morning easier:

Set out your clothes: tops, bottoms, socks
Put your shoes by the door
Put a change of socks and shoes or sandals in a bag for after the race
Fill your water bottles and put them in the fridge
Put your race snacks in your waist pack
Put your bib number on your waist pack
Put your waist pack with your keys

Enjoy your day and I will see you ladies in the morning at the grocery store parking lot that faces University at 6:00 am.

Happy Walking!

Angela"

Andrea finishes her breakfast, puts her dishes in the dishwasher and goes into the living room to do her exercises. She opens her exercise booklet, just to make sure she gets them all in.

After the exercises Andrea puts on her shoes, goes out to her garage and gets her bike out. She puts on her helmet and heads out on her bike for a casual bike ride. Riding down the road she stops at a neighbor's where they are sitting out on the front porch.

"Hi Danielle!" Andrea says to the lady on the front porch.

"Hi Andrea! How are things going? Are you still training for that race?" Danielle responds.

"Yes I am. The race is tomorrow. Today is a relaxing day. The boys are at their dad's and I am getting ready for the race."

"Very cool. Let me know how you do. I can't wait to hear about it."

"Oh, I will come over and tell you all about it. Maybe for my next race you can join me. This program really helped me. The people are great too."

"Where are you headed on your bike?"

"I am just going around the neighborhood, nothing real exciting or strenuous. Then for some lunch at home. Want to join me?"

"Sure, swing by on your way back."

"I will."

"See you soon then."

"See you soon."

Andrea peddles off down the road. She rides the outer circle of the complex, then in the inner circle, up in the front of the complex by the neighborhood pool, and then she rides back by Danielle's.

"Hey! I am headed home," Andrea shouts out to Danielle on the front porch.

"I'll be right over!"

Arriving home, Andrea puts her bike in the garage, goes inside, opens the front door, and then gets the pasta salad out of the refrigerator. She's getting everything set on the table when Danielle arrives.

"Hey! I'm here!"

"Come on in! I am in the kitchen."

Danielle enters the kitchen, "looks good. What all is in the salad?"

Andrea smiles, "a little of everything: diced ham, diced salami, diced pepperoni, diced mozzarella cheese, shredded pizza cheese, finely ground Parmesan cheese, mini farfalle or bow tie pasta and Caesar Italian dressing. I have some on the side in case you want more dressing."

"It looks delicious. Can't wait to try it."

"Thanks. What do you want to drink? I have Phyzix Tropical, Phyzix Acai Berry, Phyzix Zero, berry energy, and water. I also have Phyzix Energy Stix Natural Citrus or Mixed Berry to mix in water."

"Wow, quite the selection. I will go with the Phyzix Zero. I love the flavor, it reminds me of Squirt."

"Alright, do you want a glass of ice with it or just out of the can?"

"Out of the can is fine with me."

"Here's a can for you and one for me."

After taking a few bites of the salad Danielle says, "this is really good! This dressing is different. I like it. I'll have to get me some."

"Yes, I use whatever dressing sounds good when I am looking at the dressings. This is one of my favorites, but it is hard to find."

"Awesome. I will keep an eye out for it. Oh yeah, I got my shipment yesterday and I have started on my supplements. I really like mixing so many of them into a smoothie. It does make things easier. The only one I don't mix in is my fish oil. Next up is the exercise part."

"I can help you with some of the exercise. It'd be great to have you join me in the training program. I am planning on continuing with my training with Angela. She's at the Fitness for Life gym. I figure I'll train with her and then join the training program for the 10K next year. I love how I feel now that I am walking and exercising. I'll get you a copy of the exercises. I do them every day. It has really helped."

"That would be great. I need something. Can you take a guest to the gym? I'd love to try it."

"I don't think I can, because I haven't joined yet. I am sure that Angela could do something though and if she can't there's a really nice saleslady there named Jessie. I am going on Saturday, come on along and we'll see what they can do for you."

"I can do that. Let me know when you go to leave, and I'll come along."

They finish up their salad, Andrea puts their dishes in the dishwasher and they go out on the porch with their drinks.

"Wait here and I'll go get my exercise booklet. I have it in the living room," says Andrea and she goes to get her exercise booklet.

Returning with the booklet, she sets down next to Danielle and opens it, "here's the booklet of exercises that I was telling you about. Each page has the exercise description and a couple of pictures on it. I have found it really easy to follow. I use it every day, even though I know the exercises, I use the booklet to keep me on track and make sure I don't forget to do any of the exercises. I'll ask Angela if we can get you a copy of it."

"This is nice. I could follow these. That'd be great if I could get a copy of them."

After thumbing through the exercises Danielle says, "well, I must be going. I am sure you have things to do today to finish getting ready for tomorrow."

"Yes, I do have stuff to do, but glad we could talk. I'll see you soon."

"See you soon" and Danielle walks towards home.

Andrea goes back inside and takes her exercise booklet with her. She goes into the living room, sits down on her reclining sofa and turns on the tv. She turns her favorite channel on and relaxes for a few hours with her feet up.

The afternoon passes quickly and when Andrea looks at the time on her phone she discovers it's time for dinner. She gets up, goes into the kitchen and fixes herself a bowl of the pasta salad and a glass of strawberry water with ice. She then takes the bowl and glass into the living room to watch more of her favorite channel and eat dinner at the same time.

When she's finished with dinner she takes her dishes, puts them in the dishwasher, starts the dishwasher and goes back into the living room. Andrea checks her email, reads the email from Angela again and then she posts on Facebook about her race in the morning and how she is nervous. She gets lots of responses to her post encouraging her that she can do it and "you got this!" Scrolling through she sees that many of her friends are doing one of the races in the morning. Andrea leaves encouraging messages for her friends.

After her movie on the Hallmark Channel finishes she goes in the kitchen for some dessert. She sits on her front porch with her glass of chocolate milk and a bowl of strawberries with angel food cake. The sun is just peaking above the tree line in the west. She enjoys the sounds of the crickets in the nearby field.

Andrea thinks to herself, *I am so excited. I cannot believe I am doing my first race tomorrow. Do I have everything together? I will check on that list when I go inside.*

Looking down at her watch she sees that it's time to go in and put everything together for the morning. Andrea picks up her dishes, goes inside, puts her dirty dishes in the dishwasher, and runs up the stairs to get her things together. Andrea lays her purple tank top, black spandex shorts, purple sports bra, white Wright socks and black underwear out on her dresser. She also checks her phone and sets her alarm, two of them, so she will not be late.

Next, she grabs her sandals and puts them in a cinch sack. Andrea goes downstairs with her cinch sack and places it next to the door along with her shoes. She goes into the kitchen and fills her water bottles, one with plain water and the other with strawberry water. After she puts them in fridge she gets her race snacks together, which are a small bag of sport jelly beans and a mini size Payday bar. Her waist pack is on the counter and she puts her snacks in the pack. The goodie bag from the expo is also on the counter. Taking her bib number out of the bag she attaches it to her waist pack and then gets her keys from the key hook and sets them with her waist pack on the kitchen table.

Andrea sighs in relief that everything is together and goes upstairs to enjoy the relaxing hot tub. She turns the tv on that is mounted above the hot tub and watches a show on her favorite channel. Her show finishes and Andrea, gets out of the tub, dries off and goes to bed. She is ready for her big day tomorrow.

Chapter 22: Race Day

Andrea wakes up to the alarm on her phone going off at 5:00 am. She gets right out of bed and gets dressed. Andrea is thankful that she laid out her walking outfit last night. All dressed she is ready for a quick breakfast. Andrea goes down to the kitchen for her smoothie made of chocolate whey protein, banana, cocoa, peanut butter, and her supplements including Phyzix MD Multivitamin Plus and Phyzix MD Just for Her. On the kitchen table is her waist pack, she takes her small bottles from the refrigerator and puts them in their holder. One quick trip to the bathroom and she is ready to leave for her first race.

After putting on her shoes she grabs her waist pack, which has her bib number attached to it, and smoothie, heads out the door and drives to their meeting location. It's still dark outside, as the sun hasn't come up yet.

Andrea thinks to herself *wow, this is my first race. I am so excited to get there. Am I prepared? Of course, I am. I did all my homework. I kept up with the ladies in my group for our group walks. I have my smoothie, water and strawberry flavored water to keep me going until after the race. I will be with my group. It's going to be just like a group walk, but with a lot more people. The boys are going to be at the finish line for me. Eeeekkkk, I am so excited. I am scared, what if I fall? What if I can't make it? What am I talking about? I got this! I will do awesome! My group will be there for support. Ok, I've got this. I will do awesome! Hey, I see Angela's car. Yes, someone is here as early as me.*

Angela is sitting in her car as Andrea pulls up next to her. Andrea takes a big deep cleansing breath, picks up her waist pack and exits her truck to go over to Angela. Angela gets out of her car and opens the back hatch. She has some bananas and water.

Angela asks Andrea, "so are you excited?"

"Oh yes and nervous and scared, everything combined," she replies.

"That's ok. Everyone is their first few races and some are always like that before any race. You've done your homework and we've all done great during the group walks. You'll be fine." Angela encourages her.

Kim arrives, and Vickie pulls in right next to her. Denese and Doree ride together and pull in next to Vickie. Karin pulls up next to Kim and Sharon is the last to pull in.

Kim shuts her trunk and it pops back open. It does this a couple of times. She checks but doesn't see anything in the way. Vickie says, "take your purse out."

Kim takes her purse out and the trunk closes. She pulls the keys out of her purse and switches them with the keys in her pack. Places her purse in the trunk and this time it closes.

"How funny! I mixed up the keys. They look the same," Kim says.

"I have the same type of key and figured that was the problem. It's nice that they have keys now that won't allow you to lock them in your vehicle," replies Vickie.

"Ok, we are going to walk over to the pharmacy and use their restroom. It'll be our last chance to use an indoor restroom until after the race. Once we get across the street we will just have port-a-johns. Make sure you have your bib number on you or your waist pack. Everyone should have their waist pack with their bib number, beverages, snacks, identification, money and car keys. If everyone is ready, we can get going," Angela says to her group of ladies.

"Ready!" every replies.

Angela closes the hatch on her car and they all walk over to the pharmacy.

They enter the pharmacy and walk to the back where the restrooms are. Being that there are two single person restrooms they use both. While they are taking turns using the restroom the line grows behind them with others that will be doing one of the races. Everyone has taken their turn in the restroom and the ladies walk out of the pharmacy to the intersection where they wait for the light to change so that they can safely cross the divided road.

The traffic light turns and the ladies along with a group of other racers cross the divided road and walk down the sidewalk path that leads to the main entrance of Black Forest, where the race will start and finish. At the main entrance they wait for the traffic director to motion them across.

The traffic is starting to pick up with vehicles coming in from three different directions plus all the racers. They group crosses the main entrance and goes up the hill towards to the tents and port-a-johns. The ladies walk along the portable fencing barricades to the start/finish line where there is a banner across the timing pad on the ground. They go to the side of the banner that says start.

"Alright ladies let's take a group selfie with the start banner in the background," says Angela.

After their group selfie the ladies walk around talking to various friends that they are finding in the start/finish area.

A few minutes later there's an announcement, "Welcome to the Oakland Races! The start of the half marathon is in 10 minutes. Half marathoners, please get to your corral that matches your bib color."

Angela and her group of ladies walk over to the fence by the bleachers, so they can get a good view to cheer on the half marathon runners and walkers.

There are thousands of people around the start/finish area: runners, walkers, family and friends. "Welcome to the Oakland Races! Thank you to all of the runners, walkers, sponsors and volunteers. We are going to kick off our races with the singing of the national anthem by Riley," says the announcer.

Riley sings a rendition of the national anthem that gives everyone goosebumps. The crowd claps as he finishes the national anthem.

"All right half marathon runners and walkers are you ready?"

"YES!" they shout loudly.

"Get set…" and the air horn goes off to get the runners and walkers started. Everyone lined along the fencing that goes all the way to the entrance road is clapping and cheering them on.

"As soon as we get all the half marathon runners and walkers across the start line 10K runners and walkers, please line up according to your bib color."

Angela and her group of ladies walk over to get in line for the port-a-johns. They each have 3 people in line ahead of them. The line goes quick enough that they make it back to the fencing along the start/finish line before they announce the 10K taking off.

"10K runners and walkers we will be starting in 5 minutes!"

"MOM!" Andrea hears her boys yell to her. They come running up to Andrea with Michael walking behind them. Cooper and Carson give her a big hug. "Good luck mom!" the boys say to her.

"We'll be in the bleachers watching," says Michael.

"10K runners and walkers, are you ready?" shouts the announcer

"YES!" the runners and walkers yell back.

"Get set!" and the air horn goes off for the 10K. The runners and walkers take off down the driveway lined with people clapping and cheering them on. "5K runners and walkers, it's your turn to line up in your corral by bib color."

Andrea gives Cooper and Carson a hug. "Good luck mom," they tell her.

Andrea and her group of ladies walk to the corral with the colored flag matching their bib's color. The ladies take selfies while waiting for the official start of their race.

"5K runners and walkers, are you ready?" shouts the announcer

"YES!" the runners and walkers yell back.

"Get set!" and the air horn goes off for the 5K. The ladies walk on the side of the driveway closest to the fence and bleachers.

Cooper and Carson yell, "GO MOM!" and are clapping as they walk by them.

Vickie and Andrea are at the front of their group and walk down the driveway to the sidewalk path located between the road and the trees.

Vickie says, "let's go single file while others pass us. It's time for arms down."

The route goes to the corner of the grassy area and turns to the right where it continues along the outside of one of the parking areas to the road that leads into the campus. All along the route there are people cheering, clapping, and ringing cow bells for the runners and walkers.

Kim and Denese move to the front of the group and everyone is two by two since there is room on the road to spread out. At the first left they go left and head towards Black Forest Hall and its courtyard where there are volunteers with water.

"Water?" the volunteers ask as runners and walkers go by, while others are clapping.

"Great job!" and "Looking good!" some people are shouting as the runners and walkers go along.

Angela's group takes their water bottles out of their waist packs and gets a drink.

The route continues through the courtyard and out to the roundabout where the path goes through the trees and over the bridge. On the other side of the trees they continue along to the next left and take the road to the parking area. Here, the route veers away from the road.

Once back onto the road they continue to the section of campus that has parking by the lower soccer fields. This leads to a hill and they go up to the upper soccer fields and get to a stop sign. At the corner there are more volunteers handing out water.

"Water?" they ask, and others are clapping and cheering.

Angela and her group are all staying close together, like they did during training. As they get to the corner they follow the route to the right. At the next stop sign they turn right and this is the longest straight away that leads them to their final turn and the finish line.

"This training program has been great," says Kim.

Denese replies, "I agree. I am going to miss it. We need to have regular walks as a group."

"Yes, we do need to continue on," Andrea chimed in.

"I, too, have enjoyed our walks and would like to continue," Vickie says.

Karin says, "I will be sad if we don't get together for walks after today."

"I agree," both Doree and Sharon agree.

"I am glad to hear all this, and I can help you ladies with continuing on. We can talk about doing a 10K in the fall," Vickie says to the group.

As they get closer to their last turn Vickie and Andrea take the lead in the group and they pick up their pace pulling away from the group. They are the first to go around the turn to the right and up the hill to the finish line where Carson and Cooper are standing by the fence. "GO MOM!" they are yelling.

Their dad is standing right next to them taking pictures as Vickie and Andrea go past them and cross the finish line. The announcer announces their names as they go across the finish line. "Andrea Jo Walker from Oakland and Vickie Haus from Oakland."

Following a few seconds behind them is Kim and Denese. Doree and Sharon are next with Karin and Angela bringing up the back of the group.

After they cross the finish line there are people there to hand them their finishers medal, which they take and then proceed to the finish line goodies of apples, bananas, chips and water. Carson, Cooper and Michael meet Andrea at the open gate area at the end of the finish line goodies area. The boys give her a hug and say, "we love you mom! Great job!"

The group of ladies, Carson, Cooper and Michael walk over to the post-race celebration tent. Michael takes the boys to find something to eat and drink while the ladies go over to the free pizza and beverage line.

The boys go over to the BBQ Pit table where Cooper orders, "I want the pig candy pizza and root beer." Pig candy is a candied bacon topping.

Carson orders, "I want the macaroni and cheese with root beer."

Michael orders last, "I'll have the ribs and root beer."

He pays for their order and tells the boys, "go sit at the table right there" pointing to one that is empty, lots of chairs and close by him.

Vickie and Andrea walk over with their pizza and beverage to the table where Carson and Cooper are sitting. Kim, Denese, Doree, Sharon, Karin and Angela come over to the table with their pizza and beverages. A couple minutes later Michael walks over to the table with food for Carson, Cooper and himself.

Angela stands up and says, "Ladies, I want to thank each of you for a wonderful training season. It's been great getting to know each of you. You have finished your first 5K walk. Now you need to set your next goal. What race will you work towards? Will you do a bunch of local races? Get them paid for and on your calendar. Not only is it cheaper to sign up ahead of time, you will go to the race if it's already paid for. It is way too easy to sit at home when you wait to register until the morning of the race. You all have each other's email addresses and phone numbers. As you ladies mentioned during the race, you want to continue walking together, please do so. I can help you with training for a 10K if you like. I am always ready to help you achieve your goals. Keep an eye out for next year's training program and other training programs in the area. This will keep you going. Thank you again." The ladies all clap for Angela.

"Whoever wants to walk, just let me know. I can either bring the boys with me or with enough notice I can have their dad watch them for me," Andrea comments.

Vickie replies, "how about continuing on our Thursday group walks?"

"Yeah," they all reply.

"Ok, well I would love to continue with you ladies if you like and coordinate various places to meet," Angela joins in.

"I would love it," Andrea replies.

The rest chime in, "yes, we'd love it."

They finish their pizza and beverages. Michael along with Carson and Cooper finish their food and beverages as well and pick up their stuff. The boys give Andrea a big hug and kiss. "Bye mom!" they both tell her. Then Michael walks back to his truck with the boys.

Andrea and Vickie stay while the others get up and leave.

Vickie says, "it was so nice that Michael came with boys."

"Yes, it was. He's been very supportive. Plus, anytime I am out training on my own that means he gets more time with them, which they all like."

"That's awesome. So, what do you think about training for the 10k? I think you can do it."

"I'd love to do, especially if it's with a group. I found it much easier to walk with the group then by myself."

"Yes, it is much easier with a group. I walk by myself, but it's normally when going up to the grocery store for a few items or I'll walk home from a restaurant in town and Harvey will drive."

"That's awesome. I was looking at the maps of the 10K and the half marathon. They look challenging, especially the half marathon. It goes up Tienken."

"They are challenging, and I highly recommend them for your future. In the fall there's a 10K race in some orchards north of here that would be fun."

"I will look at it and get it on my calendar."

Vickie looks at her fitness watch and sees that she needs to get going home. "I need to head for home. Ready to go?"

"Yes, let's go." Andrea replies. So, Andrea and Vickie pick up their stuff and walk back to their vehicles.

"I had a great time this training season. We'll have to walk again soon," Andrea says to Vickie standing next to her truck.

"I agree. I'll email you and let you know my schedule."

"Have a great day!" Andrea replies.

"You too!"

Chapter 23: After the Race

Andrea arrives home after her successful completion of her first 5K walk. She parks her truck in the garage and goes inside. She sets her stuff down on the kitchen table. Andrea's legs are feeling heavy like soaked bath towels after sitting down in the celebration tent and then driving home.

She goes into the living room and starts to do her exercises that she had been doing during her training. Andrea starts out on the floor and lays back to do the supine spinal twist and lays there and falls asleep for 30 minutes. She opens her eyes, looks around, chuckles out loud and says to herself *I can't believe I laid down to stretch and fell asleep.*

Pulling her knees up to her chest and then rocking up to a seated position with her legs crossed, Andrea sits up. After a couple minutes she puts her hands down on the floor in front her, props herself up on her hands and uncrosses her legs to get into a position of being on her hands and knees. She jumps her feet back to have her legs out in a plank position, slowly she walks her hands back to be in a downward dog position. Andrea keeps walking her hands back to where she is in a forward fold and vertebrae by vertebrae stands up.

I am impressed I got up off the floor without falling over, Andrea smiles, chuckles and heads upstairs for a very well deserved hot tub time. *I can't believe how hard these stairs are. She thinks to herself. When I get to the top of the stairs I get my reward of a nice hot tub.* Andrea arrives at the top of the stairs and gives a huge sigh of relief that she has made it.

Walking into her room she just drops all of her clothes on her way to the hot tub that is in her bathroom. In the bathroom she turns on the light over the hot tub, pushes a button to retract the hot tub cover and pushes another button that gets the jets going full blast.

The next button brings up a 24" television screen, Andrea nods and thinks to herself *I am glad I paid extra for that.* The television is already set to the Hallmark Channel.

The movie playing on the television is one of Andrea's favorites, Christmas Lodge. Andrea slides into the hot tub to enjoy the movie, the bubbly hot water and some well-deserved alone time.

Hot tub time comes to an end when the movie ends. Andrea pulls herself up out of the hot tub by putting her hands up on the side and places her feet one at a time on the step inside. Andrea is able to turn and sit on the side so that she can pull legs up and swing them around to put her feet on the purple rug and stand up. On the stand by the hot tu b is her favorite purple robe. She puts it on and enjoys its comfortable and familiar feel. Before leaving the bathroom, she presses the buttons that turn off the jets, puts the television away and moves the cover back into place.

As she walks through her bedroom she picks up her planner, a pen and her laptop and walks down the stairs to relax on the couch. Sitting on the couch, she puts the footrest up, has her laptop on her lap, her planner and pen are on the big puffy arm rest. Andrea sighs while thinking *What a great morning. I finished my first 5K. My boys were at the finish line. I met some great friends. Do I do the fall 10K?*

On that note, she turns on the laptop, clicks on Google Chrome, clicks on runmichigan.com and starts searching for her next 5K race. Andrea checks the races on the website calendar with her planner. She picks out one race a month, registers on-line for it and puts it in her planner. Included in her races is the 10K that is in October.

Andrea sets her laptop aside and goes out to the kitchen to get herself a nice big glass of strawberry flavored water and ice cubes. While she is in the kitchen she also picks up some peanut butter crackers and takes them back to her spot on the couch.

It's time to sit and enjoy having done such a great accomplishment. She has her next races scheduled and is going to continue walking for 45 minutes on 3 days a week and doing her stretching exercises every day.

Before being able to relax though she sets her laptop back on her lap and sends an email to her group that says, "Thank you for all of your encouragement during this training program. I will join you all for walking. Let me know when you ladies want to walk."

Clicking the send button, she sets the laptop on the couch. Andrea leans back on the reclining couch with the foot rest up, clicks the television remote and begins to enjoy her favorite station.

Appendix 1 Training Schedule

This is the schedule that Andrea follows in this book.

Week #	Sun	Mon	Tues	Wed	Thurs	Fri	Sat
1					15 min Walk	Stretching	15 min Walk
2	Rest	15 min Walk	Stretching	Rest	20 min Walk	Stretching	15 min Walk
3	Rest	15 min Walk	Stretching	Rest	25 min Walk	Stretching	15 min Walk
4	Rest	15 min Walk	Stretching	Rest	30 min Walk	Stretching	15 min Walk
5	Rest	20 min Walk	Stretching	Rest	30 min Walk	Stretching	15 min Walk
6	Rest	20 min Walk	Stretching	Rest	45 min Walk	Stretching	20 min Walk
7	Rest	20 min Walk	Stretching	Rest	60 min Walk	Stretching	20 min Walk
8	Rest	20 min Walk	Stretching	Rest	60 min Walk	Stretching	20 min Walk
9	Rest	20 min Walk	Stretching	Rest	35 min Walk	Stretching	20 min Walk
Race Week	Rest	20 min Walk	Stretching	Race Day	Rest	Stretching	20 min Walk

Appendix 2 Training Schedule B

This schedule has a race that is on a Saturday, as many races take place on Saturdays.

Week #	Sun	Mon	Tues	Wed	Thurs	Fri	Sat
1					15 min Walk	Stretching	15 min Walk
2	Rest	15 min Walk	Stretching	Rest	20 min Walk	Stretching	15 min Walk
3	Rest	15 min Walk	Stretching	Rest	25 min Walk	Stretching	15 min Walk
4	Rest	15 min Walk	Stretching	Rest	30 min Walk	Stretching	15 min Walk
5	Rest	15 min Walk	Stretching	Rest	30 min Walk	Stretching	15 min Walk
6	Rest	20 min Walk	Stretching	Rest	45 min Walk	Stretching	20 min Walk
7	Rest	20 min Walk	Stretching	Rest	60 min Walk	Stretching	20 min Walk
8	Rest	20 min Walk	Stretching	Rest	60 min Walk	Stretching	20 min Walk
9	Rest	20 min Walk	Stretching	Rest	35 min Walk	Stretching	20 min Walk
Race Week	Rest	20 min Walk	Stretching	Rest	20 min Walk	Stretching	Race Day

Appendix 3 Exercises

The next pages have the descriptions and pictures of the exercises that Andrea does for stretching. They are just one exercise per page.

Squat with a Reach

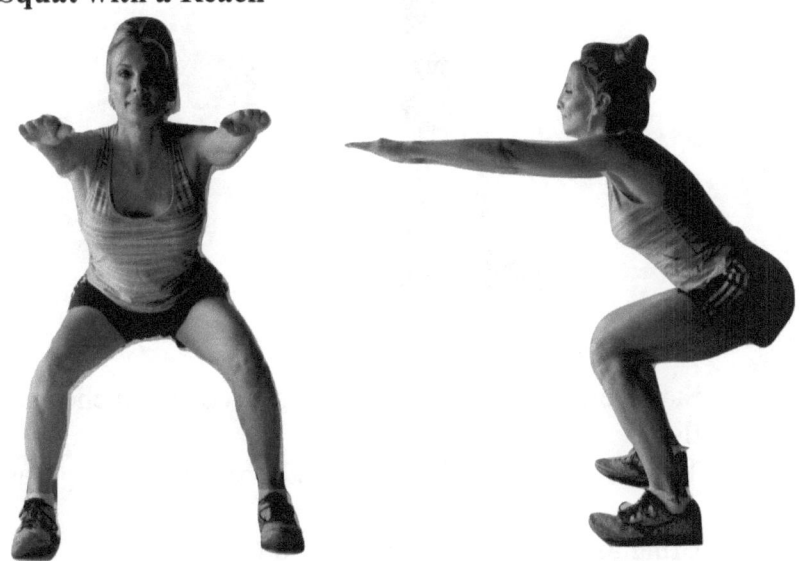

In a standing position
* feet wider than shoulders
* keep upper body tall
* squat by sticking your butt back
* at bottom of squat reach both hands forward
2 sets of 10

Single Leg Shoulder Press

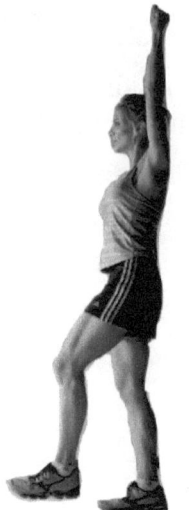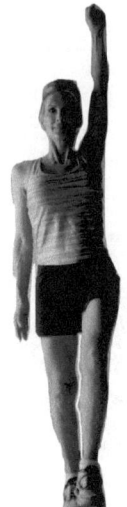

* Stand on right leg with left leg a couple inches off the floor
* Take left hand, make a fist and press fist as high as you can
* Bring arm down and place foot on floor

Repeat 12 times each side

Rapid Reaching

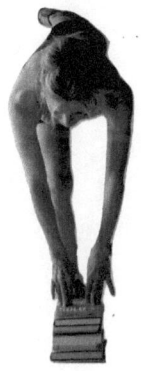 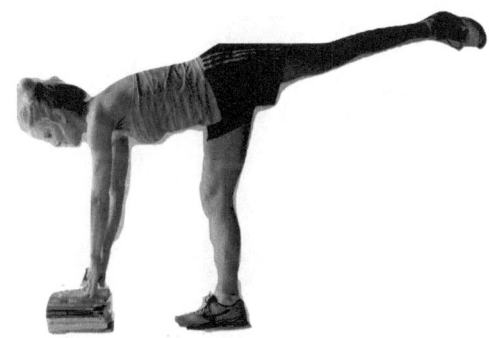

Place a small stack of items such as books on the floor in front of you

* Stand on your right leg
* Bend at the hip, keeping your upper body straight
* Reach with your right hand to touch the stack of items
* Reach with your left hand and alternate each hand 12 times

Repeat standing on left leg

Warrior II

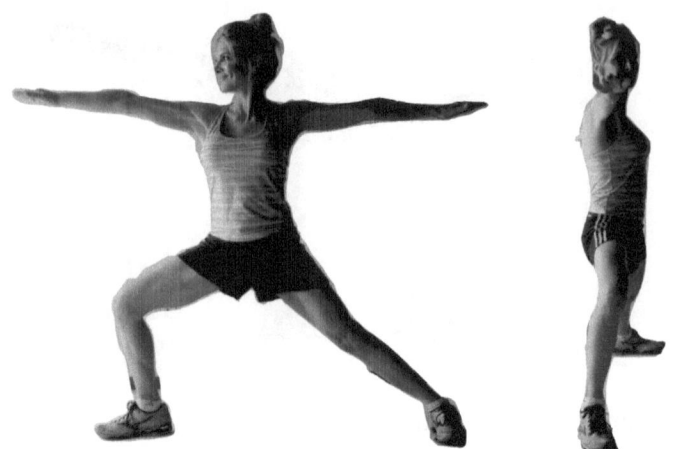

Stand with your feet shoulder width apart and toes on both feet facing forward

* Turn your right foot to the right while turning your body to face right
* Raise your arms out to your sides
* Bend your knee but make sure you can look over your knee and still see your toes
* Press your feet apart but don't move them
* Gaze over your right middle finger
* Take 4 deep breaths

Repeat with the left foot

Walker's Arms

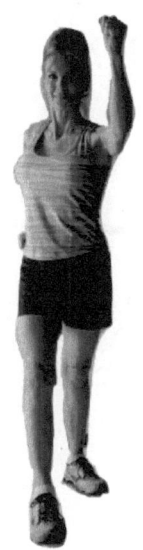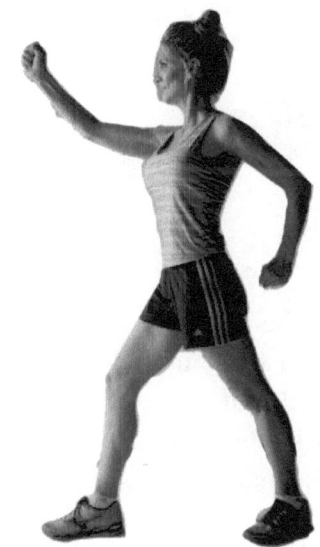

Stand with your right foot forward
* Suck in your stomach
* Bend your arms at a 90^0 angle
* Move arms forward alternately, known as pumping your arms
* Do this for 20 forward movements for each arm

Switch feet and repeat

Plank

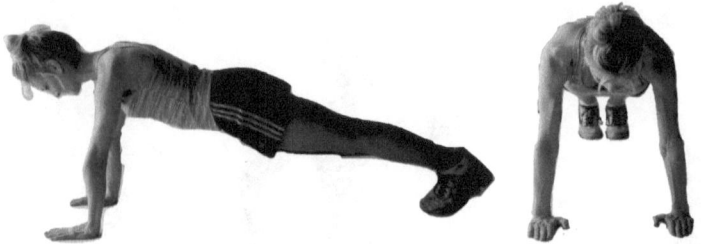

* Get down on the floor on your hands and knees
* Straighten your legs out and stay on your toes
* Keep your back flat
* Hold in your stomach
* Hold for 15 seconds
* Relax

Repeat for 20 seconds

Super Hero

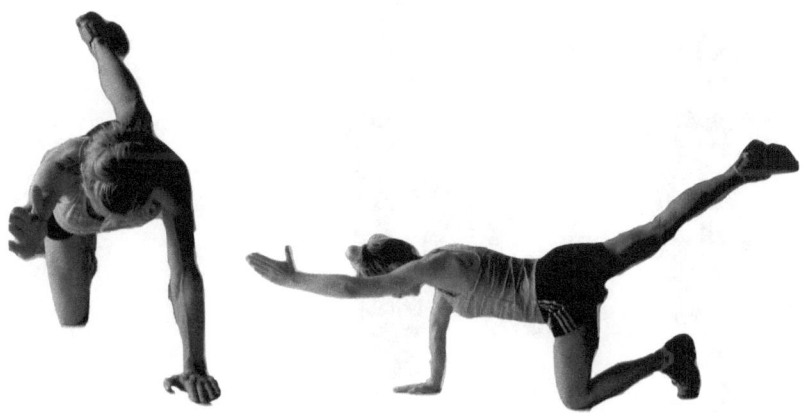

On the floor, get on your hands and knees
  * Make sure your hands are directly under your shoulders
  * Make sure your knees are a hip width apart
  * Extend your right arm out in front
  * Extend your left leg out behind
  * Hold for 20 seconds
  * Switch to your left arm and right leg
Repeat 5 times

Walking Knee Hugs

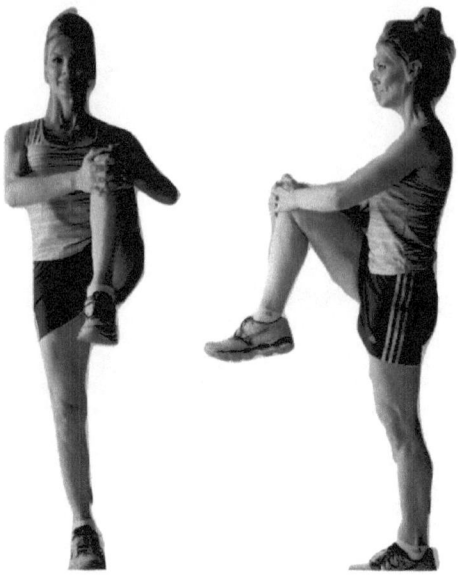

*   Walk forward with your right leg first
*   Bring up your left knee hugging it to your chest
*   Alternate knees
10 knee hugs for each leg

Triangle

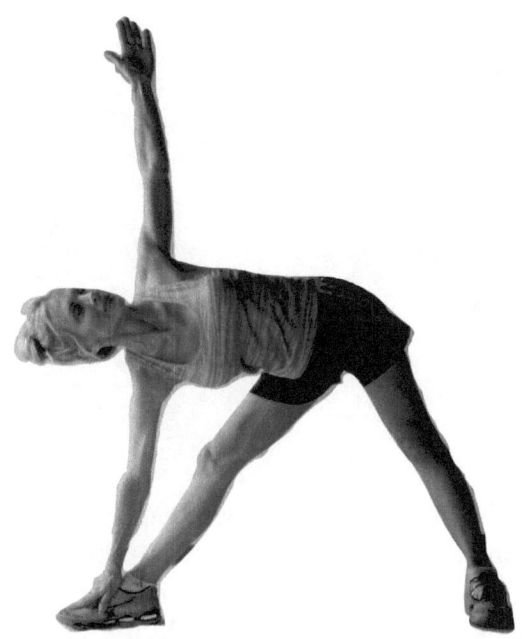

Stand with your feet shoulder width apart and toes pointed forward

* Bring arms up into a "T" shape
* Turn your right foot to the right
* Bend at the waist
* Reach your right hand to your right foot
* Turn head to look up your left arm, keep arms straight
* Take 5 deep breaths
* Rise up
* Repeat on your left

Repeat 5 times

Revolving Forward Bend

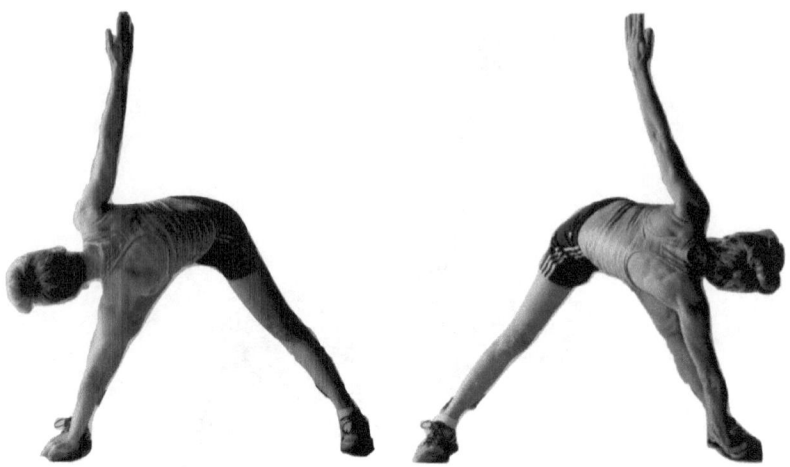

Stand with your feet shoulder width apart
* Bend forward at your waist to a 90^0 angle
* Reach both hands to the floor
* Walk both hands to your right foot
* Lift your right arm towards the ceiling
* Look up at your right hand
* Hold for 5 deep breaths
* Lower right arm
* Walk both hands to your left foot
* Lift your left arm towards the ceiling
* Look up at your left hand
* Hold for 5 deep breaths
* Lower left arm
Repeat 10 times

Downward Dog

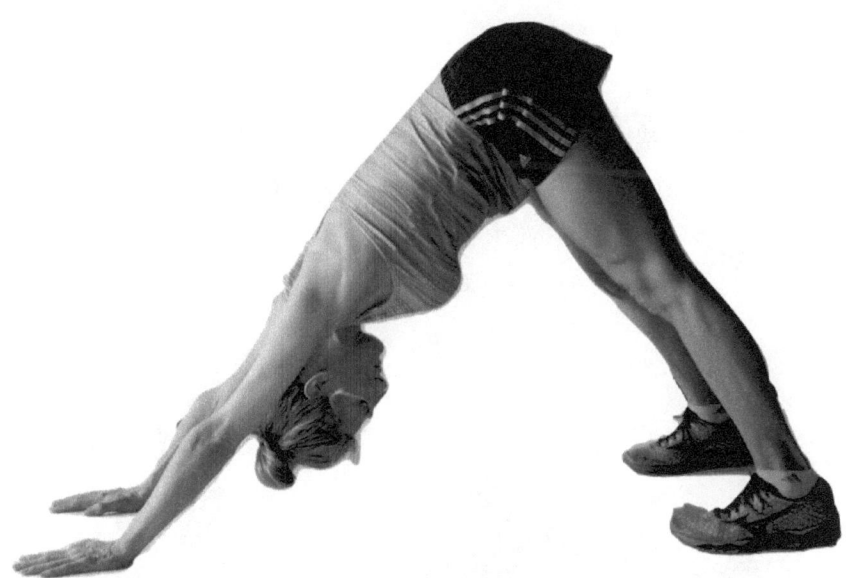

On the floor, get on your hands and knees
* Make sure your hands are directly under your shoulders
* Make sure your knees are a hip width apart
* Curl your toes under
* Lift your hips up and back
* Straighten your legs
* Hold for 5 deep breaths
* Relax
Repeat

Supine Spinal Twist

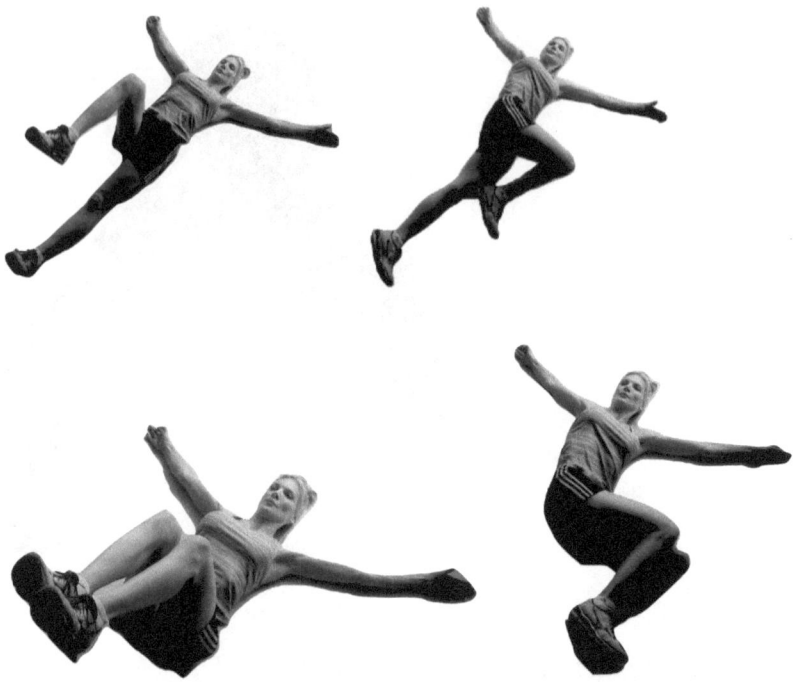

Lay down on your back
* Bring your arms out to a "T"
* Bring up your right knee to a 90^0 angle and drop it to your left side
* Hold for 5 deep breaths
* Bring your right knee back up and lay it down

Repeat with your left leg going to the right

You can also do this with both legs at the same time and go to the right and then to the left.

Thank you to Jenn Paul for being the model for the exercises. Please visit Jenn at jennpaulfit.com. Photos taken by Mandy Jo.

Appendix 4 Recipes

Andrea's Smoothie

<u>Ingredients</u>

Phyzix MD Daily Pro Chocolate whey protein – 1 scoop

Banana

Natural unsweetened cocoa – 1 teaspoon

Extra crunchy peanut butter – 2 tablespoons

Unsweetened coconut milk – 1 cup

Water

ice

<u>Directions</u>

Cut up banana, put in blender

Add 1 cup unsweetened coconut milk

Add 1 teaspoon natural unsweetened cocoa

Add 2 tablespoons extra crunchy peanut butter

Add ice to fill remaining space in blender

Add water to top of fill point of blender

Blend completely

❖ You may also add any dietary supplements to the blend

Author is not a chef and does not actually measure things when she cooks.

English Muffin Pizzas

Ingredients

English Muffins – 1 pack

Pizza cheese – 1 small bag

Pizza sauce – 1 small jar

Pepperoni – 1 small bag

Directions

Preheat oven to 375

Spray cookie sheet with non-stick spray

Separate English muffins into halves and place on cookie sheet, crust
    sides down

Spread pizza sauce on the English muffin halves

Sprinkle pizza cheese over the pizza sauce

Add pepperonis onto the pizza cheese

Sprinkle pizza cheese over the pepperonis

Place cookie sheet in oven

Watch for cheese to melt completely

Take cookie sheet out of the oven

Place English muffin pizzas on plates and serve

Enjoy!

*Author is not a chef and does not actually measure things when she
cooks.*

Scrambled Egg Skillet

Ingredients

Mushrooms – 1 small jar

Butter – 1 tablespoon

Minced garlic – to taste

Ham – 4 oz diced

4 eggs

Unsweetened coconut milk – ½ cup

Canadian steak seasoning – to taste

Directions

Chop up mushrooms, if not already

Add butter to skillet

Sprinkle minced garlic over mushrooms, according to your liking

Stir periodically while they cook

Dice up ham, if not already

Add ham to mushrooms and mix together

Crack eggs into medium bowl, whip eggs together

Add ½ cup unsweetened coconut milk to eggs, whip together

Sprinkle Canadian steak seasoning, according to your liking

Pour egg mixture over the mushrooms and ham

Let cook for a few seconds

Mix together the eggs, mushrooms, and ham

Cook until desired doneness of eggs

Author is not a chef and does not actually measure things when she cooks.

Pasta Salad

<u>Ingredients</u>

Diced ham – 4 oz

Diced salami – 4 oz

Diced mozzarella cheese – 4 oz

Shredded pizza cheese – 4 oz

Ground parmesan cheese

Mini farfalle or other small shaped pasta – 1 lb

Caesar Italian dressing or other oil-based dressing you like

<u>Directions</u>

Cook pasta according to box directions, rinse with cold water until cool

Dump pasta into a large mixing bowl

Dice ham, if not already, and add to bowl

Dice salami, if not already, and add to bowl

Dice mozzarella cheese and add to bowl

Dump shredded pizza cheese into bowl and mix thoroughly

Sprinkle parmesan cheese over salad according to taste and mix

Add dressing according to taste and mix, can always add more

Author is not a chef and does not actually measure things when she cooks.

Appendix 5 Products

These are products mentioned that Andrea uses and where you can get them to use them.

These products are all available at www.bonvera.com/10364

Phyzix MD Daily Pro – Dutch Chocolate Vegan

The protein is an all-natural pea and rice protein.

It does not contain wheat, gluten, yeast, soy protein, animal or dairy products, fish, shellfish, peanuts, tree nuts, egg, artificial colors, artificial sweeteners or artificial preservatives.

It supports protein metabolism, cardiovascular health, gastrointestinal health, antioxidant systems and provides essential micronutrients.

Also available in French Vanilla.

Phyzix MD MultiVitamin Plus

Balanced nutrients include calcium, magnesium, zinc, copper, vitamin C, vitamin E, bioactive folate, vitamin B12, B vitamin complex, beta-carotene and trace elements.

It supports a stressful lifestyle, foundational wellness, health for those with poor nutrient intake and is a basic "insurance" for wellness.

There are 120 vegetarian capsules.

It does not contain wheat, gluten, yeast, soy protein, dairy products, fish, shellfish, peanuts, tree nuts, egg, artificial colors, artificial sweeteners, or artificial preservatives.

Phyzix MD Just for Her

This is 120 vegetarian capsules.

It supports balance of the female hormone cycle and ease common symptoms associated with PMS and menopause.

It helps clear up acne.

It supports hot flashes and helps with sleeping through the night.

It also supports leg cramps, less flow during menstrual cycle and women trying to get pregnant.

Does not contain wheat, gluten, soy, animal or diary products, fish, shellfish, peanuts, tree nuts, egg, ingredients derived from genetically modified organisms (GMOs), artificial colors, artificial sweeteners, or artificial preservatives.

Phyzix MD Omega Max

This is fish oil that is certified and comes from Norwegian waters, no mercury, lead or PCBs.

There are 60 fish gelatin softgels.

It is in the monoglyceride form and is the highest bioavailable on the market.

It does not contain wheat, gluten, corn, yeast, soy protein, dairy products, shellfish, peanuts, tree nuts, egg, ingredients derived from genetically modified organisms (GMOs), artificial colors, artificial sweeteners, or artificial preservatives.

Phyzix MD Energy Stix – Natural Mixed Berry or Natural Citrus

There are 30 stix packets.

These transform your water into a great-tasting, revitalizing energy drink.

Does not contain wheat, gluten, yeast, soy protein, animal or dairy products, fish, shellfish, peanuts, tree nuts, egg, ingredients derived from genetically modified organisms (GMOs), artificial colors, artificial sweeteners, or artificial preservatives.

It does contain electrolytes, antioxidants, herbs, amino acids and B vitamins

Phyzix – Acai Berry, Tropical, or Zero

An efficient, natural energy supplement that is formulated with fruit juice and naturally occurring caffeine from green coffee beans.

Tropical contains coconut water concentrate

Increased mental focus and improved physical activity

Appendix 6 Post Walk Goodie Suggestions

Ideas for what to snack on after your walk

Green seedless grapes

Sliced strawberries

Water

Watermelon slices

Small juice boxes

Boxes of raisins

Fruit snacks

Cider slush

Mini cupcakes

Chocolate milk

Apples

Bananas

Appendix 7 Places

Some of the places used in the book are real places. Here's where you can find them.

5-1 Diner
51 S Washington
Oxford, MI 48371
248-572-7600
5-1diner.com

Bauman's Running and Walking Shop
1473 W Hill Rd.
Flint, MI 48507
810-238-5981
www.werunthistown.com

The Bavarian Inn Restaurant
Michigan on Main Bar & Grill
713 S Main St.
Frankenmuth, MI 48734
800-228-2742
bavarianinn.com/dine

The C-Pub Bar & Grille
2325 Joslyn Rd.
Lake Orion, MI 48360
248-390-3974
kingscourtcastle.com/index.php/cpub

Yates at Canterbury
2375 Joslyn Ct.
Lake Orion, MI 48360
248-48-9203
www.yatescidermill.com/canterbury

About the Author

Mandy Jo has been training men and women to walk various distances for over 13 years. During those 13 years she completed many races herself over 100 - 5K's, 11 - 10-mile, 17 half marathons, plus a marathon.

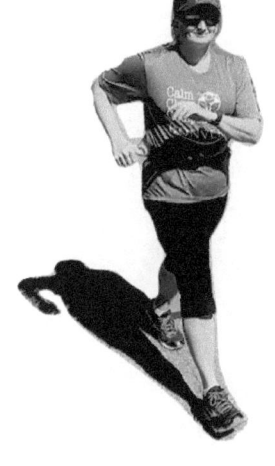

Mandy Jo also had running clubs for elementary students while her younger son was in elementary school. The goal of the running club was not solely running, but to keep moving.

While training others and herself, Mandy Jo, went through a divorce and raised two young boys, the younger one turned a year old during her first training program and the older one was seven years old. Mandy Jo's younger boy turned 1 during her first season of training for herself. After being a trainee, she switched to be a trainer.

You can follow Mandy Jo online.

facebook.com/mandyjo0830
Instagram @mandyjor830
Twitter @mandyjo830

mandyjo.us

Author photo taken by Rick Squires.

Speaking/Exercise Engagements

Mandy Jo is available for speaking/exercise engagements.

Group types

Churches

Community Groups

Schools

Businesses

Topics

Kick off your 5K training program

Get your employees moving

Help your group train for a 5K

Exercise/Stretching breaks at conferences

For more details and to schedule, please contact Mandy Jo at mandyjo@mandyjo.us

Books by Mandy Jo

Mandy Jo has more books coming in the Adventures in Walking series.

On the road to 10K

Half Marathon Bound

It's a Marathon, not a Sprint

For updates on the books, join us at facebook.com/mandyjo0830

www.ingramcontent.com/pod-product-compliance
Lightning Source LLC
Chambersburg PA
CBHW061253280526
45784CB00002B/744